Your
Pregnancy
Companion

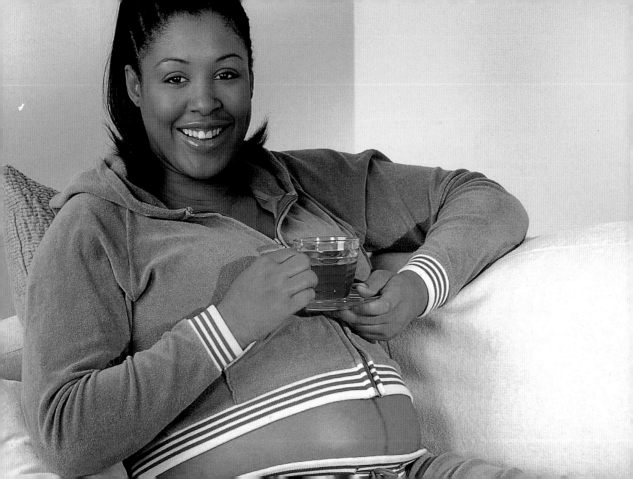

Your Pregnancy Companion

Sheila Lavery & Pippa Duncan

CARROLL & BROWN PUBLISHERS LIMITED

First published in 2009 in the United Kingdom by
Carroll & Brown Publishers Limited
20 Lonsdale Road
London NW6 6RD

Designed by John Casey and Emily Cook

© Carroll & Brown Limited 2009

Parts of the text previously published in *Meditations for Your Pregnancy* by Sheila Lavery and Pippa Duncan in 2000

A CIP catalogue record for this book is available from the British Library.

ISBN 978-1-904760-73-3

10 9 8 7 6 5 4 3 2 1

Reproduced by Rali S.A., Spain
Printed and bound in China by Leo Paper Products Ltd

Contents

Foreword

If you are thinking about having a baby or are already pregnant, you will find it invaluable to have a source of vital information in a easily accessible form as well as a place in which you can keep track of important dates, contact details and tasks completed. Designed to accompany you when you are out and about, at work, play, or travelling, *Your Pregnancy Companion* can make pregnancy worry and stress free by telling you all you need to know about, for example, what you should be eating, how much you should be exercising, whether your lifestyle habits need adjusting, what you can expect from your antenatal care, how to cope with your changing body and the expected side effects of pregnancy and much, much more.

Often as you will go about your daily activities, you'll find that some guidance would be helpful. You may, for instance, need to know whether a particular dish is safe to eat, or that something you are feeling is 'normal' or whether an exercise option is recommended. Because the book is small enough to carry with you, you can find out what you need to know without having to wait until you get home to consult a larger book or contact your healthcare advisor. And it makes interesting reading when stuck on a train or bus in the rush hour.

The text contains the most up-to-date information in a non-technical form, organised under helpful headings. Many helpful illustrations are included and a great deal of useful information is found in easily digestible charts. Diary and contacts pages are provided, which should prove invaluable as reminders when you're on the go, and there are handy checklists for shopping and packing.

Since pregnancy is a natural condition, not an illness, the emphasis throughout is on using non-medical means, where appropriate, to ease complaints and ensure safety. Special pregnancy meditations scattered throughout the book are effective ways to help you deal with stressful situations and to enable you to become closer to your baby.

How to use this book

Your Pregnancy Companion has been designed to make vital information on all aspects of conception, pregnancy, labour and delivery easily accessible.

Prior to trying for a baby, you should read through the pre-conception chapter to find out whether your diet, form of contraception or lifestyle habits need adjusting to ensure a successful conception.

Once pregnant, and wanting to know, for example, what you should do and what you can expect to happen, simply turn to the chapters on the first, second and third trimesters, where you will find all the necessary information plus ideas to try to alleviate problems. Make sure you use the diary pages to record the dates of your antenatal visits and tests.

As your due date approaches, you will find vital information on hospital routine including the different pain relief options in the chapter on labour and delivery. Here, too, are handy checklists of what to take to the hospial for yourself and your baby, as well as what supplies you need on hand when your baby comes home. There's also a place to record important contact details.

Date/Time	Place	Procedure

Important phone numbers

Birth partner	
Doula	
Doctor/midwife	
Hospital	
Taxi	
Relatives	
Maternity nurse	
Nappy service	

Labour aids

- ❏ A favourite small ornament to focus on
- ❏ Calming music that you have used before
- ❏ Comfortable cushions for support
- ❏ An aromatherapy scented handkerchief
- ❏ An atomiser water spray to freshen your face
- ❏ A flannel or sponge to cool you down
- ❏ Mirror to watch baby emerge
- ❏ A book or magazine to take your mind off labour if your contractions slow down
- ❏ Food and snacks to keep you going
- ❏ Water or juices to keep you hydrated
- ❏ Extra cushions to prop you up
- ❏ Lotion or powder for massage
- ❏ Cold and warm packs for back relief

Hospital needs

- ❏ Toothbrush, toothpaste and mouthwash
- ❏ Toiletries
- ❏ Hairbrush, clips and bands
- ❏ Dressing gown, nightgowns and underwear
- ❏ Maternity sanitary pads
- ❏ Breastfeeding supplies: nursing bra, breastfeeding pads, purified lanolin for nipples
- ❏ Watch with a second hand for timing contractions
- ❏ Change for telephone calls, parking and snacks
- ❏ Mobile phone
- ❏ Camera or video equipment
- ❏ Food and drink for your birth partner
- ❏ Slippers and heavy socks for cold feet
- ❏ Changing bag, nappies and baby clothes
- ❏ Birth announcement cards, address list and a pen
- ❏ Baby book for footprints and signatures

Going home essentials

- ❏ Loosely-fitting clothes, including comfortable shoes
- ❏ Bag for carrying home gifts and hospital supplies
- ❏ Infant car seat
- ❏ Going home outfit for your baby: vest, nightgown or all-in-one suit, socks, shawl and a sleep or pram suit, if cold
- ❏ Nappies and baby wipes

Introduction

NATURAL AIDS FOR PREGNANCY

If you're planning a pregnancy, or you're pregnant already, you're embarking on one of the most creative, most inspiring experiences of your life. It is also one of the most challenging. Being pregnant or undergoing fertility treatments can mean that you experience frequent radical changes to your mood and energy.

Once you conceive, you'll want to make the most of your pregnancy, so you need to learn to listen to your body, to respect your feelings, to pamper yourself and to nap when you need to (without feeling guilty). You'll also want to discover what you can do to overcome problems without resorting to medications or other intrusive methods.

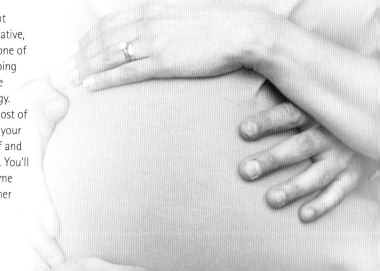

Women who suffer from pre-existing medical conditions or who are taking prescribed medications need to be closely monitored by their doctors to ensure that their treatments don't pose a risk to a developing baby, but all women need to be careful about taking over-the-counter drugs, being immunized or travelling to areas where disease may be present.

It is essential that you ensure your body provides the safe haven your baby needs to develop healthily. The first twelve weeks are particularly important, as this is when your baby's major organs and body systems are formed. Since women may not always know exactly when they fall pregnant, it is vital that they – and their partners – begin to make changes in the preconception period.

Throughout this book, you'll find the advice you need to ensure this safe haven – particularly the natural approaches that can overcome common pregnancy side effects and complaints. This chapter offers some background information on recommended techniques. Most can be safely and successfully used by anyone if the guidelines are followed, but meditation, for example, requires some practice to be truly effective. If in doubt about anything, however, do not hesitate to discuss it with a therapeutic practitioner or your healthcare provider.

Food and eating

At no other time is your body and its demands changing so obviously. Respect your body: listen to it and consider how you are going to nourish and nurture the tiny baby blossoming inside you. Don't make drastic changes to your diet but continue to develop a healthy attitude towards food instead. Now is the time to focus on the quality of what you eat and to include foods that will strengthen your health and that of your baby. Fresh food contains many beneficial nutrients. Try out new foods rather than trying to deny yourself.

A home-cooked meal on a daily basis is one of the greatest gifts you can give yourself and your baby. Cooking a meal is nourishment in the purest sense and will send a direct message of love to your baby. If you sit down to eat and have your meals at the same hour each day, you will find yourself more secure, stable, balanced and satisfied.

Your appetite may wax and wane, especially in the early months, but it usually picks up and then becomes ever bigger. To lessen mood swings related to blood sugar highs and lows, choose sugar-free jams, juices and biscuits. Also, try natural sweeteners such as rice

Top pregnancy foods

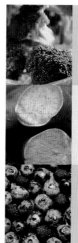

Broccoli For folate, calcium and antioxidant vitamins A, C and E. Stimulates the body's detox systems. Vitamin A is especially important in the first trimester.

Sweet potatoes For vitamin C and folate, fibre and carbs. Choose deep red fleshed varieties for higher amounts of nasty-zapping beta-carotene (it also protects skin from sun damage). Eat with cereals to double iron absorption.

Berries Raspberries and blackberries, blueberries and cherries are rich in folate, vitamin C and phytonutrients (such as anthocyanin and ellagic and phenolic acid) that are strongly antioxidant.

Avocados Rich in folate, vitamins B6, C and E, potassium, monounsaturated fats and antioxidant alpha-carotene. Folate offers up to 70 percent protection against defects to a baby's neural tube.

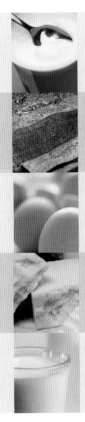

Natural yogurt More calcium than milk (a quarter of your daily requirement in one pot). Also high in zinc, protein and even fibre. Calcium is especially imprtant between weeks 4 and 6.

Organic beef The choice for B vitamins, highly absorbable iron, zinc, and of course, protein. One of the richest sources of choline. Zinc protects against low birthweight and birth defects.

Eggs Packed with minerals and more than 12 vitamins. The chromium in the yolk can ward off first trimester nausea.

Hard cheese Good eating for calcium and vitamin B12, protein, fat and carbs. B12 safeguards a baby's developing brain and nervous system.

Milk All the qualities of cheese but with vitamin D and extra Bs. A bottle of organic a day contains your entire daily recommended intake of omega-3 fatty acid. If you can't get organic, semi-skimmed has almost as much calcium as full fat.

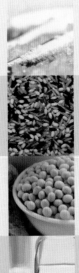

Oily fish Small fish. such as herring, mackerel and organic or wild salmon. are the best source of brain-boosting omega-3 fatty acids. They also contain valuable amounts of iron, calcium and zinc, B and D vitamins and protein.

Wholegrains The real thing: with the bran and germ come fibre and nutrients stripped out in the refining process, including antioxidant lignan and other necessaries for healthy gut flora. Always choose organic.

Chick peas Contain the antioxidant and immune-stimulant saponin as well as folate, fibre, iron and essential protein for vegetarians. Eat with a source of vitamin C for maximum absorption of iron.

Olive oil Rich in antioxidant phenolics and vitamin E as well as oleic acid to boost the development of an unborn baby's brain and nervous system.

Seeds and nuts Packed with the nutrients needed to nurture germination and new life, they include antioxidant ellagic acid and lignans, selenium, magnesium and vitamin E, protective phytic acid, plus omega-3 fats to boost brain development.

syrups, barley malt, fruit juice and maple syrup to keep you feeling calm and balanced.

When cooking, try to steam, roast or bake but if you have to fry, be sure to use unrefined oils such as olive, sesame, sunflower or safflower, which are light and easy to absorb. If you want to season food, choose unrefined sea salt over the refined table variety. Sea salt has all the trace minerals intact and will be easier to absorb.

Food choice

Eating foods that are 'whole' or that are closest to their natural states are the healthiest options for you and your baby. Eating highly processed foods or those full of chemicals creates toxicity in the body and can adversely affect your baby's development.

Rice, barley, millet, oats, corn and wheat contain both the seed and the fruit of a cereal. Each little grain is packed with energy and B vitamins, and provides you with strength and stamina. To ensure that you benefit from their goodness, include wholegrains in risottos, soups and stews, porridge or home-made biscuits; prepare couscous and bulgar wheat, and eat wholewheat pasta and breads on a regular basis.

Begin to develop a taste for fish and vegetable-quality protein such as beans, tofu, seitan and tempeh instead of meat; fish especially is rich in fatty acids vital to your baby's development. Vegetable protein is easy to absorb and assimilate. Beans and bean products are rich in essential vitamins and minerals, as well as providing slow-release energy.

Eating a wide variety of fruit and vegetables is very important. When selecting produce, look for foods that are grown locally and organically. Organically grown foods are free of toxic chemicals and give you stamina and vitality. Eating fresh vegetables on a daily basis helps you to feel more satisfied with your meals and they are an ideal complement to wholegrains.

Many different types of sea vegetables – nori, wakame and kombu, for example – are extremely valuable as they filter important minerals – iron, calcium and zinc – into the body. They also help to discharge toxins and fat.

Meditation

This simple technique, practised daily, can have significant benefits within weeks. Meditation involves concentrating on a single thought, word, image or activity and this enables you to withdraw from sensory influences, forget past or future and disregard all outside activity. The result is that mind and body are calmed and re-energised. Meditating twice a day for fifteen to twenty minutes is the most effective way to reap the rewards.

Try to establish a pattern by meditating at the same time every day: if you miss your usual slot it is often difficult to find another during the day. Most people find first thing in the morning, before getting involved in the day's activities, and early evening, but not just before bedtime when you may be too energised to sleep, convenient times. Try to meditate when you are feeling alert and rested. You also should abstain from smoking, eating or drinking caffeinated drinks or alcohol for an hour beforehand as these can all interfere with your mood.

Bear in mind the following

✓ Make yourself comfortable, but not so comfortable that you fall asleep.

✓ Sit in a relaxed upright position, not slumped or rigid, but so that your spine is straight and your breath can move freely.

✓ Aim for balance and 'openness' in your posture. Do not cross your arms or your legs. If sitting on a chair. Unclench your fists and rest a hand on each leg, preferably with palms facing upwards.

✓ Choose a posture that you can hold for ten to twenty minutes.

Places and positions

Try to sit in a special place that you can associate with meditation. Keep it clear of clutter and introduce a vase of flowers or a special picture as a focus. You also could use an essential oil vaporizer to scent the air with an aroma such as frankincense, which slows and deepens the breath and is conducive to meditation.

Find a position you can hold without becoming restless, and that will stop you from slumping or being too rigid. The following are suitable for any stage of pregnancy, but experiment until you find one that works for you.

Lotus position

It is traditional but by no means essential to sit in the lotus position, which symbolises balance and provides the body with a firm base. A few Westerners find this position easy to maintain and feel it encourages a state of relaxed awareness and mental clarity, but others find it impossible to master. The half lotus, shown here, may be easier to hold during late pregnancy).

Supported by a cushion

Sit cross-legged on a large, firm cushion tilted slightly forwards, stopping you from slumping in the small of your back. Various wedges, benches and special meditation cushions are available, but a cushion or pillow is perfectly adequate. Don't fold your arms across your body, but sit with your back erect and your shoulders back and down, opening up your chest cavity so you can breathe freely.

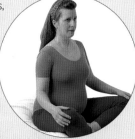

In an upright chair

If you prefer not to sit on the floor, you can meditate sitting in a straight-backed chair. Resist the temptation to sink into the nearest couch or armchair, as this will encourage you to slouch and make you feel drowsy. Sit with your feet flat on the floor, about shoulder width apart, and use a cushion or pillow to support your lower back. Rest your hands in your lap or on your knees. If, as your abdomen becomes larger, you find this position a bit cramped, try sitting closer to the edge of the chair and spread your feet a little further apart.

Lying down

The 'corpse pose' is great if you find it hard to relax. But beware: it is very easy to fall asleep in this position! Lie on your back, preferably with a mattress or folded blanket beneath you and allow the tension to flow out of your limbs by letting them sink into the floor. As your pregnancy progresses, you may prefer to lie with a pillow beneath your head and your feet and lower legs propped up on a chair, or alternatively on your side. Eventually you should be able to meditate in any position – sitting, standing, walking or lying down.

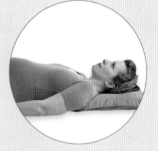

Relaxation

This is the starting point of any meditation. Conscious relaxation relieves anxiety, which tends to 'scatter' your thoughts, and releases physical tension, which can be distracting if it causes discomfort or pain.

The easiest way to learn how to relax is to find a quiet place where you will not be disturbed. Turn off the phone, make sure you are warm enough and lie or sit comfortably with your eyes closed. Let your breathing become slow and gentle, and as you breathe out, sigh to release the tension in your body. You also can relieve specific areas of tension by focusing on each part of your body, tightening it and then letting go. For example, think about your shoulders, push them down and notice where you hold your tension. Breathe out and, as you do, release your shoulders. Begin at your head or toes and work though each body part in this way.

When you first start to practise relaxation, you may feel sleepy as your adrenaline levels drop. Try to avoid

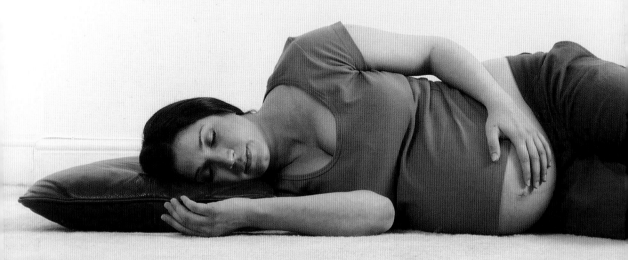

sleep by keeping your mind focused, while allowing your body to be free from tension.

When relaxing in a quiet room is not an option, you can adapt the above technique to use in an instant. Think 'relax', push your shoulders down, and as you breathe out with a long sigh, let all the tension from your head to your toes flow out with it. Another simple technique is to take three deep breaths, and with each slow exhalation feel the tension flow out on your breath as your shoulders drop and your belly softens.

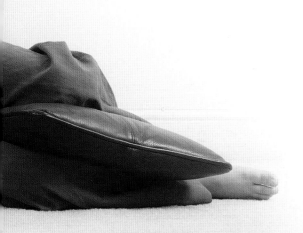

Finding a focus

Meditation involves using a single focus to still the mind and create a state of inner tranquillity. Anything that absorbs your attention can act as a focus to shut you off from other distractions, but breathing, mantras, affirmations and visualisations are most often used.

When attempting to focus your mind, however, you may find the following points help:

- Choose a simple point of focus and devote your whole attention to it. Go for five minutes at first, gradually increasing to twenty minutes.
- Do not force your mind to concentrate. Focus, but without effort. Simply decide that you will attend to one thing only and let it hold your attention, disregarding all distractions.
- When intrusive thoughts attempt to crowd in (and they will), don't try to push them away, just let them float by without giving them any importance.
- If your mind wanders, gently bring it back to your focus.
- Accept that you may not succeed at first – and keep trying!

The breath

The simplest and often the best focus for meditation is your breathing. The breath is rhythmical, balanced and natural, so observing it helps to relax the body and quiet the mind. All relaxation techniques and antenatal classes make use of breathing as a way of relieving tension and easing pain and anxiety.

One technique is simply to count your breaths. Count from one up to five, then start again at one. Try not to force or control your breath, just observe it as it comes and goes at its own pace, and feel how it moves and reverberates through your body. Relaxed breathing is not regular, so your counting should not be regular either. Try to match your counting to your natural breathing pattern rather than regulating your breath by the pace of your counting. Stay relaxed and focused. If your mind wanders, gently steer it back. Do this for fifteen minutes.

If you prefer not to count, you can simply observe the movement of your breath in your body. Sit relaxed, one hand placed flat over your navel, the other just below your breasts. Breathe in and allow it to fill the lower part of your lungs, before moving down to your abdomen. Let the air wash over your baby and expand your abdomen before moving back up to lift your ribs and spread out your collarbones. Allow the breath to flow through you, and follow it with your mind as it relaxes, clears and refreshes every part of your body with which it comes into contact. As you breathe out, do so slowly from the top downwards, deflating your ribs and then your belly, but not slumping the spine, as you exhale completely. Do this several times so that you become aware of what good breathing feels like.

Now close your eyes and continue to breathe as above, but do not follow it with your mind. Focus only on the movement of the breath in your abdomen – the way it rises and falls with every in- and out-breath. Keep breathing in this relaxed way with your concentration centred on your abdomen for fifteen minutes of the day. Regular deep breathing that expands your lungs and abdomen will help to relax you and get you into the habit of breathing well.

Mantras

Many people find the best way to achieve mental stillness is through the repetition of a simple word, phrase or sound that is used to block the intrusion of other words and thoughts. Thinking one thought repeatedly leaves no room for others to intrude, focuses the mind in one direction and frees it from the usual emotional congestion that typifies everyday thinking. The word or sound chosen for this purpose is known as a mantra, a Sanskrit term meaning 'instrument of thought'.

Some people believe the words of a mantra should have a healing or mystical effect, for example, 'God is love', but a mantra can be a word or a sound without any real meaning. Simple, meaningless or inspiring words, short phrases or sounds work best as a mantra. You could try one of these – 'Peace', 'Love', 'Relax', 'One', 'Joy', 'All is one', 'We are one', 'Om', 'Om Ah', 'Shalom', 'Allah hu', 'God is love', 'Om mani padme hum' or any other mantra of your own devising. Some words, however, should not be used as a mantra. 'Mother', for example, has too many psychological associations; similarly, 'Birth' or 'Baby' are too emotional to still your mind.

Whichever mantra you choose, you can repeat it not just during a proper meditation but throughout the day, while doing the housework, going for a walk or waiting in the doctor's surgery. The simple repetition very quickly soothes and relaxes.

When you are sitting comfortably and relaxed, focus on your mantra and repeat it over and over again. You can say the mantra aloud or to yourself. Even if you choose to say it silently, it is sometimes a good idea to say it aloud to begin with and let it become progressively quieter until it becomes a whisper and then you internalise it completely. This way you can get a feel for it. Most people find it helpful to synchronise their mantra with their breathing, saying it on every out-breath, or on every in- and out-breath. You can also say your mantra independently of your breathing. Either way, focus on the word or sound to the exclusion of everything else. If your attention wanders, simply bring it back to your mantra. Saying it aloud can help to regain your attention.

Some people find mantras too boring to focus on for fifteen to twenty minutes. If using a mantra makes your mind drift rather than focus, return to simple breath counting or try one of the other techniques described on the following pages.

Affirmations

Affirmations are similar to mantras in that they are words or phrases that can be repeated over and over again throughout a meditation. But there are also some basic differences between the two. Affirmations are often phrases rather than single words. The words of an affirmation always have meaning and the meaning is more important than the sound. They also tend to be 'tagged on' to a meditation in which you use the breath as a focus rather than being the focus themselves. Here are some affirmations you might like to try:

- Today is a perfect day
- I am (we are) happy and well
- I am peaceful
- I love how relaxed and in control I feel
- I am complete
- My beautiful baby is wanted and welcomed
- I am loving and lovable
- I love and cherish my perfect baby
- I am willing to change and grow
- All is well.

You can use affirmations to confirm and encourage changes that are taking place in your body during the relaxation process. If you tell yourself in a calm and focused way to 'Slow down' or 'I am relaxed', your body tends to respond accordingly. As your body starts to relax, repeating an affirmation such as 'I feel warm and heavy' (if you do) can help you to become more aware of the physical sensations associated with relaxation, so it then becomes easier for you to recognise when you are relaxed.

Do not think about the affirmation, just repeat it silently and continuously to yourself, while remaining focused on your breath. You can repeat the affirmation in time with your breathing, but remember the breath, not the affirmation, is your focus. If you find it difficult to combine the two, let go of the affirmation until you feel more focused and return to it later. Combining your affirmation with a visualisation (see page 22) can have even greater impact. If your affirmation is, 'My beautiful baby is healthy and well', hold an image in your mind of your perfect, healthy developing child.

You don't have to restrict affirmations to a formal meditation: you can use them whenever you need to give your mind positive instructions. For example, if you are anxiously awaiting the results of tests you could tell yourself, 'Everything is as it should be', or if you have been suffering from morning sickness you could begin your day with, 'This morning I feel happy and well.' In such situations, affirmations can have a positive effect on mind and body, but they do not produce the sort of relaxed awareness associated with meditation.

Using a visual aid

If you prefer to meditate with your eyes open, you can help to keep your mind focused by meditating on a pleasing image. The goal is to gaze at and be aware of the object, but not actively to think about it. In theory, any object will do but, like a mantra, it should be free from any psychological or emotional associations that might encourage your mind to wander.

It is traditional to use a visual tool that has some symbolic value – a lit candle, a picture, something with of a geometric shape, a patterned bowl.

By learning to visualise an object internally, you will find it easier to meditate anywhere and at any time: once you can hold an image in your mind, you can recall it at will from your visual memory. The following exercise is designed to improve your visualisation skills.

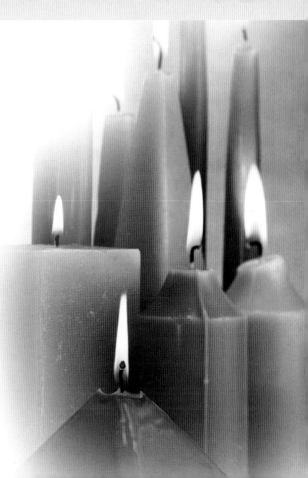

- Look at an object and absorb it visually, without attempting to memorise it.
- Close your eyes and hold the image in your mind for as long as you can without forcing it.
- When it fades, open your eyes, look again at the object, and repeat the procedure. With practice you should be able to retain at least the shape of the object to use as a stimulus for future meditations.

Visualisation

Imagining a scene can have essentially the same effect on body, mind, emotions and behaviour as perceiving that scene in reality. So picturing yourself relaxed and happy on a sun-kissed beach can actually make you feel relaxed and happy, and seeing yourself as a capable, confident mother can make you feel exactly that. Not every image has the power to do this. For greatest benefit, the image you create must be strong and you must be able to hold it for as long as you need to. You should believe in the image and be involved in it, whether it is realistic or complete fantasy. Some people find it easier to visualise than others, but you can improve your creative imagination with practice. Sit comfortably, relax and close your eyes. Conjure up an image in your mind. It could be a colour (see also page 23), a flower, a point of light or a beautiful scene in the country or by the sea – whatever makes you feel relaxed and happy. Use the image as your focus. Explore it, using all of your senses. If you 'see' yourself on a beach, feel the sun on your back, the sand between your toes, hear the waves lapping on the shore and smell the seaweed. Go for a swim, feel the water as it cools your skin, taste its saltiness, enjoy the weightlessness of your body floating in it. When you come out of the water, let the sun dry your skin, bask in its warmth and relax.

If your mind strays from details of the scene, just bring it back and continue to explore your image for twenty minutes. At the end of your meditation, gradually allow the image to fade. Bring your attention back to the room and the present. In your own time, open your eyes, stretch gently and get up.

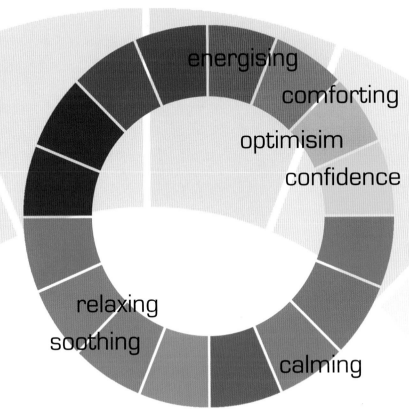

energising

comforting

optimisim

confidence

relaxing

soothing

calming

Each colour has its own attributes: red is energising and can help you overcome tiredness, ease pain or stiffness in your lower back and legs and improve circulation. It also is comforting if you feel alone or insecure. Yellow can improve digestion and concentration and foster optimism and confidence. Green is calming, reduces high blood pressure and is good for anxiety or resentment. Pale blue is relaxing, calms the nerves and soothes the emotions. It is good for insomnia, skin irritations and haemorrhoids.

Meditating with a partner

This can be particularly beneficial if you are planning or expecting a baby, as both of you share the same goal of enjoying a successful pregnancy and producing a happy, healthy child. It also can strengthen your relationship through having something else you can share, with the additional benefit of making both of you feel relaxed, more in harmony and bonded together in a special way.

A partner can lend support when your meditations seem unproductive and encourage you to practise when you may not want to. Knowing there is somebody else meditating with you can strengthen and deepen your meditation. You also can learn from shared experiences – comparing notes can reveal more about the process and help you to have realistic expectations about your achievements, although it is also important to keep something of your meditation to yourself. In some cases, focusing together on a problem can provide a solution that you may not have been able to arrive at alone.

Meditating with a partner is essentially no different from meditating alone as each person's meditation is always individual. You simply share the same space and

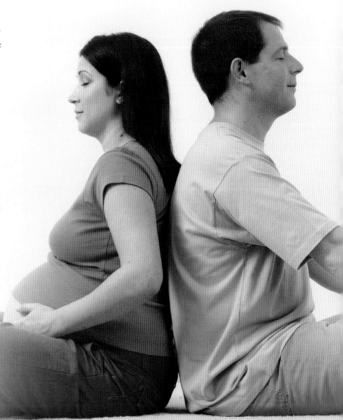

meditate at the same time. You do not need to use the same focus or aim to achieve the same goal, although this can be beneficial. For example, you could meditate together with the view to becoming a closer family. Even if your meditations have the same aim you might use different techniques – and if you share a technique such as visualisation, your visualisations will be different. Do not attempt to fit in with what your partner is doing; just do what is right for you.

What is important is that you respect each other's needs, feelings, privacy and confidentiality. Agree on when, where and for how long you will meditate so that there are no disruptions. You also should agree on details such as incense, lighting and whether one of you would disturb the other by chanting aloud or breathing noisily. Working in this way with a like-minded partner once or twice a week can be beneficial, but it does not work for everyone.

After meditating with a partner, ask yourself whether you gained something from the experience or found it restricting and unproductive. Remember, shared meditation should be mutually beneficial and involve a sense of oneness with each other. You should not feel as if you are competing with your partner, so if the experience does become competitive or demanding, go back to meditating alone.

Ending a meditation

Every session should end with a brief period of quiet rest. It is common to feel a little light-headed when you finish, so sitting in silence will help to ground you and bring your attention back to everyday life. You also could practise a simple grounding exercise.

Sit up straight and relaxed, and place your feet firmly on the ground. Breathe deeply into your abdomen and push your feet into the floor. Think of your feet sprouting roots, which grow into the ground, binding you to the spot. If you are sitting in a chair, let it take your weight and get a feeling of your bottom sinking into the seat. When you stand up, stamp your feet a few times to feel in contact with the floor.

It also can help to have a small snack or a drink when you finish meditating as this has the effect of bringing you back into reality and returning your attention to your everyday physical needs. Practical tasks have a similar ability, so you could follow your meditation by cooking or gardening.

Aromatherapy

People have been using aromatic plants and their healing oils for thousands of years to treat and soothe the whole body emotionally, physically and spiritually. Aromatherapy oils can be used in baths or showers or applied directly to the skin.

Aromatic baths

A few drops of an essential oil in a bath can revitalise and revive or calm and sedate, alleviate aches and pains and promote deep, restful sleep. Simply add six to eight few drops of the essential oil of your choice (see below) to warm water, relax and enjoy the benefits. In the shower, add a few drops of your chosen essential oil to a cotton washcloth and relish the delicious vapours while standing under the running water.

On the skin

Massage is a great way to feel relaxed and to soothe aching muscles. Essential oils are too potent to use directly on the skin, so first dilute a few drops of an essential oil in an almond oil base and then apply this mixture to your skin. Applying oil to your belly can help to prevent stretch marks and to maintain your skin's natural elasticity. A foot massage can be a great treat you can do yourself while you'll need your partner to give you a full body massage.

Oils

There are a number of oils that should be avoided during pregnancy, so check the label or ask an experienced aromatherapist for advice. Here are some oils that you might like to try.

Lavender oil is excellent for soothing aches and pains, especially in the legs and the back. It has stress-relieving, antidepressant and anti-nausea qualities and also promotes restful sleep.

Mandarin is refreshing and gentle, and counters fatigue and fluid retention.

Neroli is an extremely expensive oil but has the most luxurious scent. It is especially valuable for the regeneration of the skin and promotes healthy, clear skin.

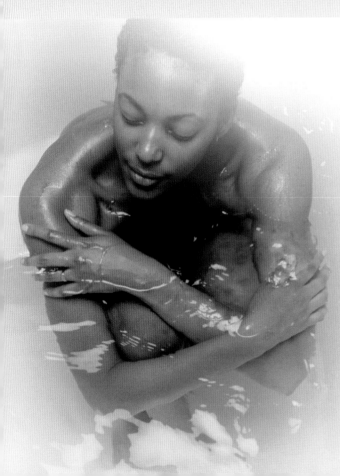

Tangerine is a cheerful oil that is beneficial for stretch marks. Its mild nature helps to calm nerves with a wonderfully uplifting smell.

Ylang-Ylang is an exquisite oil that is both relaxing and restoring. It is good for those who are tense or worried.

When buying essential oils, choose ones in dark, glass bottles, rather than plastic bottles, and do not store oils in plastic as it degrades quickly and taints the oils. Make sure you purchase pure essential oils (only these have therapeutic properties) and buy only a small amount at one time. Expensive oils are an indication of their quality; a small amount of an expensive oil goes a long way. Store your oils in a cool, dark place.

Homeopathy

This is a safe form of medicine in which remedies aim to stimulate the body to 'cure itself'. The remedies contain extremely diluted agents, which given in full strength, would produce the symptoms currently experienced. Homeopathic remedies can be made from plants and inorganic substances and are generally taken in pill form.

Homeopathy can be effective in combating minor pregnancy complaints such as heartburn, nausea and vomiting, and some women find it can help during labour. Homeopathic remedies are unlikely to cause side effects to either mother or baby, as only a very minute amount of the active ingredient is used in a specially prepared form. However, in pregnancy you should always consult a professional homeopath, as pinpointing the right remedy can be quite difficult.

Bach Flower Remedies

Developed by a medical doctor and homeopath, this therapy claims that plants contain natural 'vibrations' that can be used to restore harmony and health. There are 38 individual remedies widely available. They are not harmful and some may be useful in pregnancy – to aid relaxation and overcome anxiety, for example.

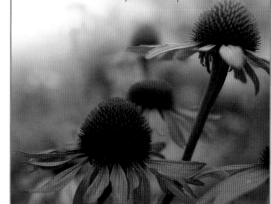

Acupressure

A non-invasive technique, this is a type of massage that aims to boost the body's self-curative abilities and can relieve pain, reduce tension, promote relaxation, rebalance the body and maintain good health. The most well-known form of acupressure, shiatsu involves using the hands, fingers and thumbs to stimulate key pressure points on the surface of the recipient's skin. In pregnancy, acupressure can be helpful in relieving nausea and then later on, may provide pain relief in labour.

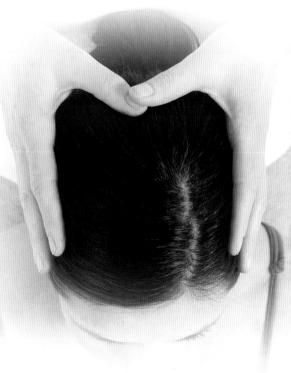

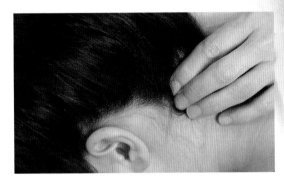

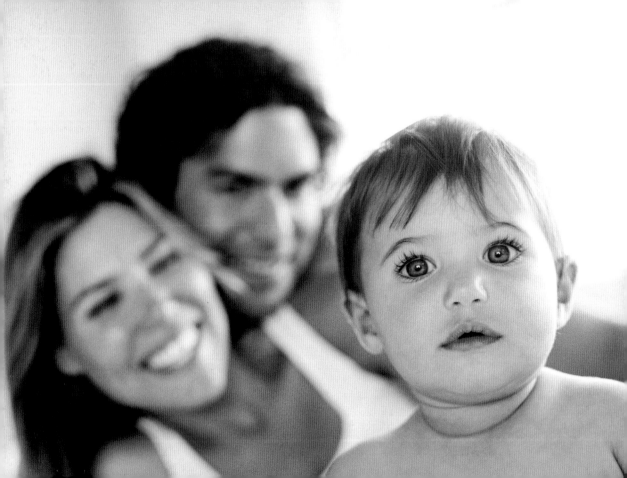

Chapter 1

A successful conception

HELPING TO ENSURE A HAPPY OUTCOME

Today we know much more about the process of conception, enjoying a healthy pregnancy and giving birth to healthy children than did past generations when "falling pregnant" was something of a mystery.

Preparation for parenthood should begin as soon as you decide that you want to become pregnant. Laying the foundations for the months ahead, both physically and emotionally, improves your chances of having a successful pregnancy and birth, a healthy baby and a happy postnatal period.

In addition to boosting your fertility by clearing your body of toxic substances and poor quality foods (see Boosting Your Fertility, below), it also is the time to clear out emotional stresses and strains and to create within yourself a state of perfectly balanced health.

Achieving balance

Emotional health, like physical health, is a prerequisite to a successful conception. Stress is thought to be a major cause of infertility. Your body responds to stress as it would to a threat, and in times of danger, reproduction is not at the top of nature's list of priorities. Emotional wellbeing is important, too, to libido and for looking ahead positively to when you are pregnant and then a parent. And if conception doesn't occur as soon as you'd like it to, being in good emotional health will help you withstand any disappointments or setbacks.

Dealing with stress

Deciding to have a baby, especially your first, is a major life change. Even happy events can be stressful and for some people, trying to conceive can take months of anxious waiting. The thought of parenthood can be daunting as well as tremendously exciting, and it is easy for both partners to feel under pressure when you want everything to go perfectly.

The most basic requirement for any process of growth and healing is relaxation and there are many techniques available. There also is a wide choice of complementary therapists who are trained in stress reduction. On a personal level, time management techniques can make life less pressured.

Managing time

Planning ahead, setting priorities, and making use of people who could help you, all will help you to achieve what you want and thus prevent you feeling anxious. Make a list of everything you need to achieve, making sure you are realistic about the time needed and including periods of relaxation and exercise. Try to organise your week so the most demanding and important chores are done when you are feeling the most alert. See if you can delegate some of the less important or less interesting chores or maybe reconsider whether they need to be done at all!

Relaxing

Some people become relaxed by sitting down with their feet up, while others need to engage in activities involving breathing and muscle control such as the

Alexander Technique, yoga or t'ai chi. Practising meditation can switch off the stress response and rebalance the body, including the hormonal and reproductive systems, so you are much more likely to become pregnant. Progressive muscle relaxation (see page 232) also helps to relieve tense muscles and induce a relaxed state.

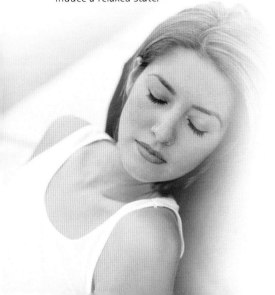

Aromatherapy

Essential oils such as neroli, sandalwood and lavender when applied to the body during a massage can induce feelings of calm. Some oils are to be avoided during pregnancy so it is best to consult a trained aromatherapist if you will be engaging in self massage.

Reflexology

Pressure points on the foot can be manipulated to bring about the relief of stress and minor ailments. Some relief can be obtained through self massage but a trained reflexologist will produce a better result.

Acupuncture

Practitioners believe that the free flow of energy, or chi, along pathways in the body is necessary for the body to be in a relaxed and healthy state. They insert fine, painless needles into areas of blockage to free up the chi. Not only has acupuncture been proven to aid relaxation but it can assist with fertility treatment and relieve side effects.

Encourage relaxation

Use this meditation when you want to

- Relax your mind and body

- Relieve the stress that can hinder conception

- Instill feelings of calm and contentment

How to practise this meditation

Sit comfortably in a quiet place and begin by relaxing your body. Focus your attention on your abdomen and breathe in all the way down to the pit of your belly. Feel it swell as you breathe in and let it sink as you breathe out. Allow your breathing to come and go as gently as possible, and with every out-breath feel the tension drain from your muscles. Keep focusing on the rise and fall of your abdomen until your breathing establishes its own relaxed pattern.

Now close your eyes, without altering your breathing, and concentrate on the word 'Relax'. See the word written in large, chunky letters in the darkness behind your eyes, and focus only on that word. As you breathe out, say 'Relax', silently or aloud or let it escape as a whisper on your breath. As you say it, see the word spread and slump in your mind's eye as if the letters were melting; then, as you breathe in, pull it sharply back into shape. Keep focusing on the word, seeing it liquify as you exhale and re-form as you inhale. Don't impose a rhythm on your breathing: allow it to find its own pace and let all other thoughts go.

mini meditation
An instant calmer

If you practise this meditation often, your subconscious mind will quickly learn to associate the word 'Relax' with the state of relaxation so that you can relax on cue. In future times of stress, anxiety, pain or discomfort, simply taking three deep breaths and saying 'Relax' on each long, slow out-breath can bring instant comfort and relief.

Getting closer to your partner

Most people want to have children together because
they love each other. It is all too easy, however, to get
overly focused on conceiving. Baby-centred lovemaking
can become more of a chore than a spontaneous act of
pleasure and passion, so be sure to keep a loving
physical relationship alive throughout your
reproductive cycle.

Mindful loving
Mindfulness is about being completely absorbed in any
activity you do. Being mindful of your lovemaking lets
you savour each moment of togetherness with your
partner and takes your mind off baby worries. Use all
your senses, emotions and thoughts to experience each
moment. This will increase your enjoyment of all that
life has to offer, strengthen your attachment to your
partner and relieve anxieties about the future.

Trying for a baby
If you've been trying to have a baby for some time, be
careful not to become too fraught. Bear in mind that
while each menstrual period may seem like your body

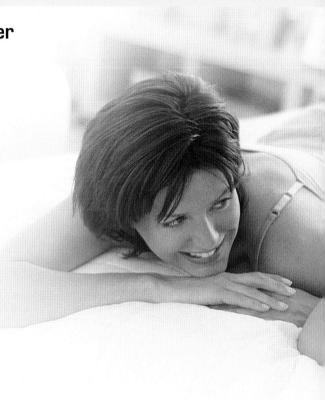

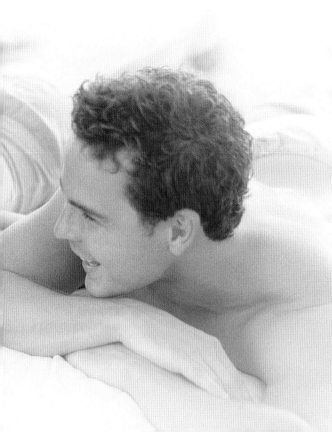

is betraying you, it also is disappointing for your partner. He may feel that his virility is being questioned, or that he is being treated like a baby-making machine rather than the man that you love.

It's important not to lose sight of the closeness between you. Focus on the fact that you are together because you love each other, and not because you would make perfect parents. Encourage that love to grow by making time for each other, appreciating each other's qualities, continuing to enjoy each other's company, and meditating to help retain a sense of calm and generosity.

Couples who meditate together claim to enjoy greater harmony and intimacy. But even meditating alone may strengthen your relationship by focusing your attention on improving yourself, rather than trying to find fault with your partner. Meditation also encourages the growth of happiness within yourself. People who are happy, tolerant and loving are less likely to be thoughtless or quarrelsome.

Become more loving

Use this meditation when you want to

- Strengthen your bond with your partner

- Increase your enjoyment of the present

- Improve your capacity to love and be loved

How to practise this meditation

Place a rose bud or any other flower bud in front of you. Sit down, relax as normal and look at the flower with half-closed eyes. Focus on it in a relaxed way and let all other thoughts float out of your mind.

Study the flower and as you become more aware of its shape, colour and beauty, imagine it growing in your heart.

Close your eyes and visualise it inside you, waiting to be coaxed into bloom by the power of love. When it does flower, it will radiate love all around you. Keep focusing on the bud and see it gradually unfold its petals and spread out, little by little, to take up the whole space of your heart. Eventually, you can see nothing else – your heart has become the flower.

The flower's fragrance is like the scent of love. It permeates all the cells and tissues of your body and wafts out through your pores. The perfume envelops you and radiates from you. Your heart is full of love; you feel loved and loving, complete and serene.

Continue to sit for a few minutes, focusing on your heart flower, enjoying its fragrance and radiance before opening your eyes.

mini meditation
In times of crisis

When you feel angry with or hurt by your partner, try the following Buddhist technique to instill love in place of bitterness. Visualise an image of yourself being superimposed on your partner and hold the image for as long as you can. You should find it difficult to stay upset when you see parts of yourself in your partner.

Adjusting your contraception

Once you have decided to try for a baby, you may think all you have to do is come off whatever form of contraception you are using. However, it is a good idea to inhibit conception (though not fertility) while you make any needed changes to your diet and lifestyle.

While you prepare for pregnancy, you need to consider whether your current contraceptive method needs changing; some forms may pose a risk to pregnancy and/or a developing fetus.

You also may want to know how long your current form of contraception may prevent your chances of conceiving. Sterilisation techniques – tubal ligation and vasectomy – are meant to be permanent and only may be reversed with surgery and even then, restored fertility is not guaranteed.

Hormonal methods vary in their effects on fertility; with some, ovulation may be extensively delayed. Barrier methods like the diaphragm and condom, however, are instantly reversible.

Certain "natural" methods – those that rely on changes to cervical mucus and body temperature (see pages 76-9), also are useful to identify particularly fertile periods, which is helpful when you are trying to conceive.

The chart on the following pages covers the various methods of contraception and their effects on fertility and risks for pregnancy. Consulting it can help you decide on the best approach but you may want to discuss the matter with your doctor.

Method	How it works	Effect on fertility	Risks for pregnancy
COC (combined oral contraceptive pill)	Inhibits the uterine lining preparing for implantation and thickens the cervical mucus so sperm are prevented from entering.	Variable. Women who have never been pregnant before can experience long delays as do women over 30 (a year or more) although many women ovulate within a few weeks, even days, of stopping the pill. Users of triphasic pills may find their fertility returns quicker than those on monophasic pills.	A greater risk of a multiple pregnancy for women who conceive while taking the pill. Although babies are not generally affected if their mothers conceived while on the pill or shortly after, it is recommended for your health to stop taking the pill 3 months before you want to conceive.
POP (progestagen only pill)	Those containing Desogestrol inhibit ovulation. Older forms thicken cervical mucus and interfere with sperm transport in the Fallopian tubes.	Traditional forms are very short-lived; fertility may return within 12 hours of a missed dose with no evidence of any delay in fertility. The new pill has a longer-lasting action and is less likely to fail.	A greater risk of an ectopic pregnancy for women who conceive while taking the traditional POP. Some women taking it have very infrequent periods, so it's possible to conceive and not realise it. There is no evidence that being on this pill in early pregnancy can damage the baby.
Injectable hormones	Inhibit the pituitary and hypothalamus so very little of the hormones that stimulate the ovaries are released. Any cervical mucus produced is infertile.	On average, fertility returns within 6 months of the last dose expiring, but can take up to 18 months, even if you have had only one injection.	Very few accidental pregnancies occur and there doesn't seem to be a risk of ectopic pregnancy or miscarriage, although babies may tend to be underweight at birth. This effect is most marked if the baby was exposed to an injection soon after conception.

Method	How it works	Effect on fertility	Risks for pregnancy
Subdermal progestagen implant	A matchstick-sized rod is inserted under the skin of the upper arm to thicken the cervical mucus and stop ovulation occurring for up to 3 years. A double rod gives 5 years' protection.	Fertility returns very quickly after removal; most women will within 7 weeks. It may take a few cycles to read fertility signals accurately.	Because it is so 99.7% effective, there have been very few true failures. Most recorded pregnancies with an implant are due to insertion after an unknown conception.
IUCD (the intrauterine contraceptive device)	Makes the uterus unreceptive to a fertilised ovum and inhibits sperm motility.	Immediate. Pelvic infection is rare if sexually transmitted infection is avoided.	More than a 50% risk of a miscarriage if an IUCD is left in place after accidental conception. If the device is removed within the first 3 months of pregnancy, there is a high chance of a successful pregnancy and a low risk of congenital abnormalities. Pelvic infection may be more severe for women using an IUCD, so it's preferable not to use one until your family is completed.
IUS (the intrauterine system)	Thickens cervical mucus so it becomes impenetrable to sperm. If fertilisation occurs, implantation is unlikely. Ovulation may be inhibited and periods usually become light.	Fertility should return within weeks after removal.	Low risk of ectopic pregnancy so suitable for women who have suffered a previous ectopic pregnancy. Risk of miscarriage if the device left in place.

Method	How it works	Effect on fertility	Risks for pregnancy
FA (fertility awareness) or NFP (natural family planning)	Changes in body temperature and the composition of the cervical mucus can signal ovulation permitting you to avoid intercourse during these fertile times.	Immediate and completely reversible. May even promote fertility by allowing intercourse to be timed for the fertile days in the menstrual cycle.	No evidence to suggest any health risks to a baby conceived accidentally.
Barrier methods (male and female condom, diaphragm, cervical cap) and spermicides used together	Prevent sperm entering the cervical canal; spermicides kill sperm.	Immediate and completely reversible.	No increased risk to babies conceived accidentally using barrier methods with spermicides.

BOOSTING FERTILITY

Doctors recommend that you increase your chances of conceiving and delivering a healthy baby by preparing for conception between three and six months in advance. This means getting your mind and body in shape by improving your physical fitness, eating a healthy diet, eschewing bad habits like smoking, drinking and drug taking, and reducing your exposure to environmental pollutants.

Getting in shape to conceive

A healthy body weight is crucial for fertility; both too low and too high a weight can interfere with the hormones needed to stimulate ovulation and as well as cause other ovulatory problems.

Overweight women have a much lower success rate for IVF. When pregnant, they face an increased risk of gestational diabetes, pre-eclampsia and miscarriage.

Underweight women, once pregnant, are at a higher risk for miscarriage or of having underweight babies or babies being born prematurely and therefore vulnerable to infection.

Professionals use the BMI (Body Mass Index) to gauge total body fat and hence the risk of fertility problems. BMI is calculated as weight (kg)/height (m) squared. For example, if a woman is 1.72 metres tall and weighs 65 kg, her BMI would be 65kg/(1.72 x 1.72m) or 22.03 (see also page 157)..

Having a healthy BMI (between18.5 and 24.9) is ideal for fertility. If you are overweight, a reduction in weight of five to ten per cent will increase fertility. You can achieve this through eating a healthy, balanced diet and exercising for at least 30 minutes three times a week.

If you are underweight, it is important to try to gain weight to come close to your ideal BMI but to do so in a healthy way (see page 48).

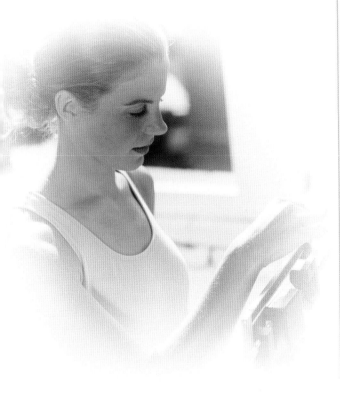

To lose weight

✓ Limit your fat consumption, especially from animal and dairy sources.

✓ Eat more fresh fruits, vegetables and low-fat dairy items.

✓ Exercise regularly including at least 20 minutes cardiovascular activity per session.

✓ You may need to change your contraceptive method.

✗ Don't lose more than 2 lbs per week. Aim for the high end of the ideal weight range.

To gain weight

✓ Eat according to your appetite and always have regular meals.

✓ Eat plenty of starchy foods and oily fish and avoid low-fat dishes.

✗ Don't over exercise especially with vigorous activities such as endurance training or running.

✗ Don't fill up on sweet and fatty foods that offer little in the way of nutrients.

Exercise options

Regular, moderate exercise (30 minutes three times a week) can improve your physical well being and mood and ensure your body is in the best shape for pregnancy. Different activities benefit your health in different ways – some build muscle, others increase flexibility – but all can be rated in terms of stamina and suppleness. Aerobics, swimming, and gymnastics for example, score high on both measures while jogging is better for stamina than suppleness and yoga increases suppleness over stamina. In terms of weight loss, aerobics, disco dancing, skipping, cycling and running burn the greatest amount of calories.

If you haven't exercised in a while, start with gentle exercises – swimming, walking, yoga – to improve suppleness, then start to add in more vigorous exercise such as aerobics, cycling and jogging to increase your stamina. You know you're building your fitness if the session leaves you slightly out of breath, causes a rise in your pulse rate and makes you sweat a little.

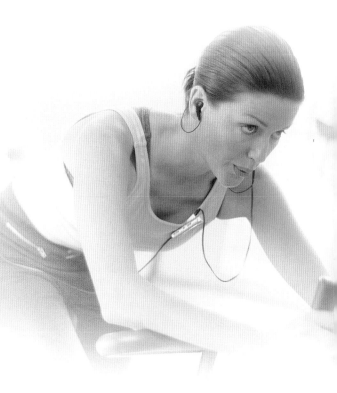

Fitness components of different activities

Sport	Muscular Strength	Aerobic Stamina	Muscular Stamina	Flexibility
Aerobic class		✓	✓	✓
Dancing	✓	✓	✓	✓
Circuit training	✓	✓	✓	✓
Walking		✓	✓	
Running		✓	✓	
Rowing	✓	✓	✓	✓
Swimming	✓	✓	✓	✓
Martial arts	✓		✓	✓
Downhill skiing			✓	
Gymnastics	✓		✓	✓
Racquets sports		✓	✓	✓
Golf		✓		
Cycling		✓	✓	

EATING TO PROMOTE FERTILITY

Ensuring both you and your partner are eating enough of the nutrients that are essential for fertility can help bring about a successful conception. If necessary, you and your partner should try to make the needed dietary improvements six months before you plan to conceive.

A fertility boosting diet must include an abundance of a wide variety of fresh foods. Fruit and vegetables provide antioxidant vitamins essential for reproductive function in men and women; milk, seafood and nuts provide zinc, needed for sperm production and healthy fetal development; meat and poultry provide amino acids, necessary for semen production; and 'good' fats provide essential fatty acids, a prerequisite for the proper functioning of the reproductive system.

The main components

A healthy diet is made up of five major groups, commonly displayed as a pyramid. In ascending order, these groups are starchy or carbohydrate foods, vegetables and fruit, dairy products, proteins, and fats and oils. The idea is that you eat more of the foods at the base and fewer of those nearer the top.

Starchy or carbohydrate foods
These foods provide energy and, if wholegrain, fibre, iron and B group vitamins. At least a third of your diet should come from this group.

Bread, breakfast cereals, potatoes, grains such as rice, wheat and oats, are all part of this group. Try to avoid refined versions as they contain less nutrients though some refined foods are fortified with certain vitamins and minerals.

A healthy balance of food

Oils and fats Limit your intake to less than 30% of your daily calories.

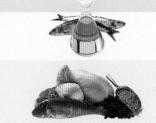

Proteins Eat 2 to 3 portions a day. A portion = 85g (3oz) meat, 115g (4oz) fish or 140g (5oz) cooked lentils.

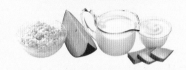

Dairy products Have 3 portions a day. A portion = 200ml (⅓ pint) of milk, 140g (5oz) yogurt or 40g (1½oz) cheese.

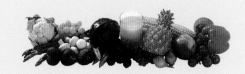

Vegetables and fruit Aim to eat at least 5 portions every day. A portion = 1 glass of orange juice, 1 piece of fruit (e.g. an apple) or 3 tbsp cooked vegetables.

Complex carbohydrates These should form the largest part of your diet. Eat 6 to 7 portions daily. A portion = 2 slices of bread, 140g (5oz) potatoes, 4 tbsp cooked rice or 6 tbsp cooked pasta.

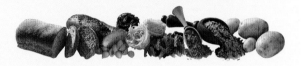

Vegetables and fruit

These contain essential vitamins, minerals and phytochemicals. About a third of your daily diet should be made up of fresh vegetables and fruit.

Eat a mix of different colours to ensure you get the maximum benefit. If you must cook them, use steam or microwave them just after preparing otherwise many of the nutrients will be lost. Fresh is best but frozen and canned are also good if fresh sources are unobtainable or past their best. Vegetable and fruit juices also 'count'.

Dairy products

An important source of calcium and other vitamins, dairy products also provide protein for women who don't eat meat. Full-fat milk, butter, yogurt and cheese are high in fat, so choose low-fat versions. About 15 percent of your diet should be made up of these foods. Make sure to keep them refrigerated to preserve their goodness. Soft and blue cheeses are not recommended for pregnancy as they may contain bacteria harmful to a baby, so it may be best to avoid them while you are trying to conceive (see also page 54).

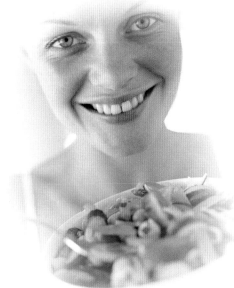

Proteins

Meat, fish, poultry, eggs, pulses, nuts and tofu contain amino acids, which are the building blocks of the body, as well as a wide range of other essential vitamins and minerals. You need only eat about three portions per day to get their benefits. However, only meat, poultry and fish contain complete proteins, so women who don't eat these foods must ensure that they eat a range of pulses and prepared vegetarian sources to get all the necessary proteins.

Fats and oils

Fatty foods provide energy, fatty acids and fat-soluble vitamins and minerals but you only need to eat a small amount of them to gain the benefits. Good sources include avocados, peanut butter, nuts and seeds, fatty fish and their oils.

Fats that are liquid at room temperature – vegetable and fish oils – are preferable to those that are solid – meat and butter.

Fibre

Found in a number of different foods – vegetables, pulses and grains, nuts and seeds – this is essential for eliminating toxins from the body, absorbing energy and maintaining a healthy digestive system.

Tips for healthy eating

✓ Eat at least 5 portions of fresh fruit and lightly steamed or raw vegetables a day.

✓ Choose organic items wherever possible, particularly milk.

✓ Bake, grill or steam to maintain essential vitamins and minerals; avoid fried foods.

✓ Have your vitamin and mineral levels checked; correct any deficiencies.

✓ Take a high quality multivitamin and mineral supplement, which contains iron, zinc, magnesium and vitamins C, E and B complex to enhance your fertility.

✓ Take 400 mcg of folic acid a day to reduce the risk of your baby developing neural tube defects.

✓ Filter all water and aim to drink two litres a day.

✗ Avoid coffee.

Fluids

An adequate fluid intake is essential; you should aim to drink about two litres per day. As much as possible of this should be water, but milk, herbal teas and fruit and vegetable juices also are good choices. Other fluids, such as carbonated drinks and those containing caffeine, can aggravate digestive problems and may result in water loss, so are best avoided. Alcohol can affect fertility (see page 60) and neither partner should drink it during the pre-conception period.

Water

Although not a nutrient, sufficient water ensures that your blood is able to deliver nutrients to where they are needed. In pregnancy, drinking water also can help prevent constipation.

Some tap water may contain toxins that can interfere with conception, such as lead and nitrates, so it's a good idea to request a report from your water supplier. If in doubt about the water's quality, drink filtered water – about eight 225-ml glasses per day.

Its important to take care with bottled mineral water as some brands contain a large amount of sodium. Choose those that contain less than 200mg per litre or buy spring water.

Coffee, tea, and caffeinated drinks

Before you conceive and during at least the first 12 weeks of pregnancy, it is recommended to avoid caffeine. Large intakes of caffeine have been linked to infertility and even moderate consumption in early pregnancy raises the risks of miscarriage and low birth weight babies. A study by The American Journal of Obstetrics and Gynaecology found more than 200mg of caffeine a day – or two cups per day – doubled the risk compared to abstainers while between two and four cups of tea or coffee a day may delay conception. The current recommendation in Britain is to drink no more than 200mg per day (see page 53).

While trying to conceive, its best to switch to decaffeinated drinks or herbal or fruit teas.

Caffeine is found also in certain cold and flu remedies, so always check with your GP or another health professional before taking any of these.

Herbal and fruit teas

Some alternatives to green and black teas include blackcurrant, blackberry, rosehip, apple, hibiscus and nettle tea. As well as being caffeine-free, these teas also can be safe and natural ways to help relieve minor ailments and aid relaxation. In pregnancy, certain herbs are uterine stimulants and should be avoided. These include ginseng, fennel, sage and peppermint.

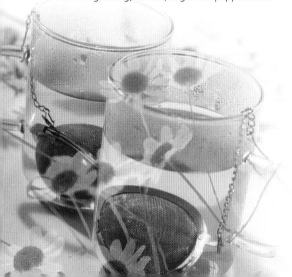

200mg of caffeine is roughly equivalent to

- 2 average cups of instant or brewed coffee.*
- 4 average cups of tea.*
- 5 cans of regular cola drinks.
- 3 cans of so-called "energy" drinks.**
- 5 50-g bars of dark chocolate; milk chocolate is about half of plain chocolate.

* The caffeine content in a cup of tea or coffee varies by different brands and brewing methods. Coffee sold in coffee shops have higher levels of caffeine. A small cafe latte in Starbucks contains 240mg of caffeine.

** A new generation of energy drinks, including Spike Shooter, contain up to 300mg caffeine in a single can. Red Bull, typically, contains 80mg.

Foods to avoid

As a general rule, overly salty, sugary and fatty foods should be eliminated entirely from your diet. They not only provide you with 'empty' calories but they can prevent you eating more of beneficial foods. Some other foods also should be avoided as they can cause infections and diseases that can result in miscarriage or problems in a developing baby.

Cheese

Blue cheeses such as Stilton, gorgonzola or Danish blue, where you can see the blue veining, or those that have a soft rind of mould such as Camembert, Brie or chevre (goat's cheese) should be avoided. The risk from these cheese is listeriosis, which is a flu-like illness but which can cause miscarriage or stillbirth (see also page 58). If the cheese is used in cooking, however, any listeria will be killed – provided the food is piping hot.

Cheeses such as cottage cheese, cream or processed cheeses, feta, mozzarella, ricotta, mascarpone and hard cheeses such as Cheddar are safe to eat. However, if you are in any doubt about a cheese's safety, the best advice is not to eat it.

Pâté

Liver and liver products are not safe to eat because of the large amounts of retinol they contain. This could cause malformations in a developing baby. Other types of pâtés such as fish, meat or vegetable varieties that you buy from the delicatessen counter could be prone to listeria contamination, a serious infection (see page 58). If they have been heat treated such as canned, or you make your own, they should be safe.

Fish

Oily fish store dioxins and polychlorinated biphenyls in their flesh and too much could harm an unborn baby. Mackerel, salmon, herring, sardines, pilchards and trout can be eaten up to twice a week in pregnancy but some large fish – marlin, king-mackerel, tilefish, swordfish and shark – should not be eaten because they may contain mercury, which could damage your baby's developing nervous system. Tuna is safe to eat but in limited amounts. You can have two fresh tuna steaks weighing about 170g before cooking or up to four medium cans (140g drained weight) of tuna per week.

Raw fish is not safe to eat as it may contain tiny worms, which are destroyed when cooked or frozen. Sushi, which is made freshly with raw fish such as that sold in some sushi bars, is not safe to eat. Most sushi available in supermarkets and some restaurants is bought in and, by law, has to be made using frozen fish. If you are in any doubt, ask if the fish has been frozen. If yes, then it is safe to eat.

Raw shellfish such as oysters or other uncooked shellfish should not be eaten. Shellfish such as mussels, prawns and crab is all fine to eat in pregnancy provided it has been cooked properly so that any bacteria or viruses it may be contaminated with are killed.

Nuts and seeds

It is a good idea to avoid eating peanuts during pregnancy if you or any family members suffer from allergies such as hayfever, asthma and/or eczema. Almonds, along with cashews, hazelnuts and Brazil nuts are tree nuts, and current advice suggests that to eat these in moderation in pregnancy is fine.

Eggs and foods made with raw eggs

It is not safe to eat foods that contain raw eggs such as home-made mayonnaise, sorbets or some desserts including tiramisu, cold soufflés or mousses as they may contain salmonella bacteria, which can cause food poisoning. Shop-bought versions of these are safe to eat, and if you are eating out and are unsure whether your meal may contain raw egg, make sure to ask. You can eat eggs cooked in any way provided the white and yolk are fully cooked.

Raw or undercooked meats

Dishes such as carpaccio and steak tartare should not be eaten and all meat and poultry dishes should be cooked until all pinkness has disappeared; this is especially important for minced meat dishes. Raw meat contains bacteria that can cause food poisoning.

Key vitamins, minerals and other nutrients

Vitamin/Mineral/Nutrient	Required for	Good sources
Vitamin A 600mcg/day*	Male and female sex hormone production. Helps to regulate the thyroid gland. Once pregnant, it is vital for baby's cell growth and weight gain.	Found as beta carotene in plant foods and retinol in dairy and meat products. Red, orange and yellow fruit and vegetables, such as mangoes, peppers and carrots; dark green vegetables, such as watercress, spinach and broccoli; and eggs, butter and cheese.
Vitamin B1 (thiamine) .8mcg/day	Converting starchy food into energy and the normal functioning of the nervous system; helps alleviate the effects of stress.	Meat (especially pork and bacon), yeast extract, whole grains, pulses and eggs.
Vitamin B2 (riboflavin) 1.1mcg/day	Energy release and healthy eyes and skin.	Milk and other dairy, yeast extract, whole grains and pulses.
Vitamin B5 (pantothenic acid) 5-10mcg/day	Functioning of the immune system and for energy release.	Whole grains, pulses, brown rice, mushrooms, yeast extract and green vegetables.
Vitamin C (ascorbic acid) 60 mcg/day	Resistance to infections and toxins, helps healing.	Most fruit and vegetables; citrus fruit, potatoes and green vegetables are particularly good sources.
Vitamin E 15-30iu/day	Hormone production and sperm function, muscle strength. Helps metabolise essential fatty acids. Muscle strengthening.	Sunflower and corn oils, whole grains, avocado, egg yolk, green leafy vegetables and peanuts.
Vitamin K 45-80mcg	Blood clotting.	Leafy green vegetables such as spinach and broccoli.
Folic Acid (folate) 400-600 mcg/day	Red blood cell formation, cell division, protein synthesis, transmission of genetic code and metabolising zinc.	Leafy green and root vegetables, chickpeas, whole grains, milk, salmon and dates.

*Recommended nutrient intake during pre-conception

Vitamin/Mineral/Nutrient	Required for	Good sources
Calcium 800-1200mcg/day	Growth and maintenance of bones and teeth, blood clotting and nerve and cell functioning.	Dairy products, soy milk, sardines, whole grains, nuts and seeds
Copper 1.2mg/day	Brain, bone, nerve and connective tissue development.	Dark leafy greens, dried fruits such as prunes and apricots, meat, nuts, rice, cocoa, black pepper and yeast.
Iodine 140mcg/day	Maintenance of normal thyroid function.	Seafood, iodized salt, dairy products and eggs.
Iron 10-18mcg	Red blood cell production, resistance to infection, helps prevent miscarriage.	Red meat (not liver), eggs, pulses, spinach and dried fruit.
Magnesium 270-350mcg/day	Circulatory system function, healthy nerves, muscles and bones.	Seeds such as pumpkin, melon and sunflower, dried fruit, bananas, milk and leafy green vegetables.
Manganese 1.4mg/day	Bone development; memory and nerve functioning.	Whole grains, seeds, yeast, bananas, eggs, and leafy green vegetables.
Potassium 3,500mg/day	Healthy fluid balance, heart muscle and nervous system functioning.	Fruit – fresh and dried, vegetables, nuts, meat, pulses and whole grains.
Selenium 100mcg/day	Resistance to infections and toxins, protects cells from damage.	Brazil nuts, red meat, fish – especially mackerel, kippers and herring, wholemeal bread, Cheddar cheese.
Zinc 30mcg/day	Maintenance of male and female hormone levels, production of semen, tissue growth and repair.	Red meat, whole grains, shellfish, seeds, vegetables and fruit.
Essential fatty acids (Omega 3, 6, 9) 700-1000mg/day	Production and regulation of sex hormones and fetal brain development.	Cold pressed oils, leafy green vegetables, fatty fish and seeds.

*Recommended nutrient intake during pre-conception

Food-related infections

Certain foods and food preparation techniques can cause problems that can affect a developing embryo, so it is a good idea to avoid these food-borne infections during the pre-conception period as well.

Toxoplasmosis

This is caused by a parasite found in raw meat and unpasteurised milk, which can lead to brain damage and blindness in a developing baby. It must be treated with antibiotics, which can be damaging during pregnancy, so its best to ensure you are safe from infection. The parasite is carried by many animals and appears in cat feces, so you must always wash your hands each time you have handled a cat or kitten and wear gloves when handling cat litter. If you do not, then you need to wash your hands thoroughly afterwards. Always empty litter trays within 24 hours.

Salmonellosis

The salmonella bacterium causes severe symptoms such as nausea, abdominal pain, diarrhoea, and fever and in severe cases can be fatal. Infection with salmonella often can be traced to eggs and chicken meat so it is recommended that you cook eggs and chicken well, avoid eating dishes that contain raw eggs, and prevent raw poultry and eggs coming into contact with other foods.

Listeriosis

This is caused by a bacteria found in many foods such as soft and blue cheeses and patés. It also multiplies at low temperatures so 'cook/chill' meals must be heated thoroughly to at least 70°C (160°F) for at least two minutes. It is also found in soil and water, and is carried by some animals. In pregnant women, the bacteria can cross the placenta and seriously affect a baby, or may cause miscarriage or stillbirth.

Good kitchen hygiene

✓ Keep a separate plastic chopping board for preparing raw meat and poultry.

✓ Cook meat, eggs, shellfish and pulses thoroughly.

✓ Thoroughly wash all vegetables and fruit, particularly those eaten raw.

✓ Set your refrigerator temperature to below 4°C (32°F).

✓ Reheat food until steaming hot for at least two minutes; throw away any left-over reheated food.

✓ Keep eggs in the fridge.

✓ Wash pet utensils separately from your own and wash your hands after handling animals.

✓ Always buy and eat food before the "sell by" and 'use by' dates listed on the packaging.

✓ Keep your kitchen and food serving area really clean. Bleach cloths and work-surfaces regularly; wash tea towels daily and don't use as hand towels.

✓ Transfer your food to the fridge as soon as possible after shopping; do not leave it in a warm place such as the office or car.

✓ Wrap or place in containers any raw meat, poultry or fish, which may drip onto other foods; place in the coldest part of the fridge.

✗ Stop eating liver, paté, soft and blue cheeses, undercooked meats and dishes made with raw egg.

✗ Do not refreeze defrosted food.

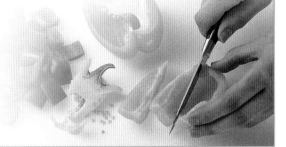

Quitting bad habits

It is well known that it is unwise to smoke, drink alcohol or use drugs during pregnancy, but these bad habits also can adversely affect fertility. Tobacco, for example, contains toxins, which, among many other harmful effects, lower levels of the reproductive hormone oestrogen in women and reduce sperm quality in men. Alcohol can depress a man's ability to perform sexually and damages sperm production; it also can increase the risks of miscarriage and still birth.

Quitting cigarettes, alcohol and drugs will not only enhance your fertility, it also will leave you in better health for pregnancy and parenthood. But giving up is rarely easy, even when you have a good reason. Habits are comforting, not necessarily because you like doing them, but because the very act of doing something repeatedly makes you feel secure. Kicking one habit can leave a huge gap in your life that you feel desperate to fill with another.

Meditation, if practised twice a day, also can be thought of as a habit, so if you use the meditations in this book, they can help you to believe that you are replacing your bad habits with a much better one that will enhance your fertility and improve the health of you and your baby.

Drinking alcohol

Couples today who are planning to start a family are advised to moderate their drinking habits. The toxic effects of alcohol can affect the ability of men and women to produce healthy sperm and ova. In the testes and ovaries, alcohol interferes with the delicate process of cell division, just as the chromosomes are being sorted and separated, a time when accuracy is so important. Alcohol causes organic brain damage to a developing fetus, as well as restricted growth, physical abnormalities, and problems of the heart, nervous system, kidneys and liver.

On average, men who drink four units of alcohol a day run the risk of having a lowered sperm count. Also, high numbers (sometimes more than 50 percent) of the sperm that they do produce can be abnormal. Alcohol depresses the hypothalamus gland and reduces the levels of stimulating hormones, which may interfere with ovulation.

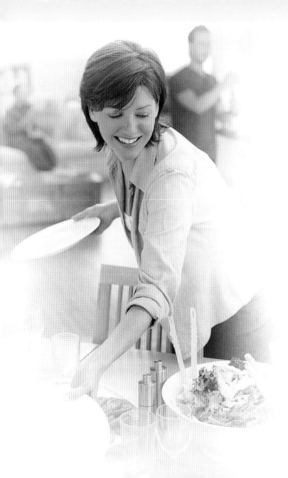

Good reasons to quit smoking, drinking and drug taking

✓ Pregnant women who smoke are more likely to miscarry, bleed during pregnancy and give birth to premature or small babies.

✓ Babies born to smokers have reduced immunity to infections in the first year and are at greater risk of cot death (sudden infant death syndrome).

✓ Children of smokers have been shown to have reduced intellectual capacity and may suffer malformations such as a cleft palate.

✓ Drinking heavily during pregnancy can cause a life-long disability called FASO (Fetal Alcohol Spectrum Disorder) characterised by mental retardation, physical deformities, and heart and nervous system problems.

✓ Certain drugs can reduce fertility and later, during pregnancy, cause fetal abnormalities or affect a woman's health. Stop using recreational drugs and consult your doctor if you take prescribed medication.

Establish healthy habits

Use this meditation when you want to

- Replace bad habits with better ones

- Reduce the stress and symptoms of withdrawal

- Purify your body

How to practise this meditation

Sit or lie down comfortably in a quiet space. Relax and start to breathe in through your nose, deep into your lungs and abdomen, and out through your mouth. Spend some time finding a level of deep breathing that feels comfortable. Close your eyes and be aware only of the movement and rhythm of your breath.

After a few minutes, visualise the air you are breathing in as the cleanest, most healing white light you have ever seen. As you inhale this purifying light, see it fill up your lungs and imagine it spreading out all around your body, cleansing and healing every cell with which it comes into contact. See it purify and protect your uterus in particular. Continue to focus on this image, while also imagining your out-breath moving up from the base of your belly. As it moves up, see it sweeping all the toxins out of your abdomen and lungs. See the old stained breath leaving your body to be replaced by the clean white light. Gradually see the air you exhale become cleaner, until it is as white as the air you are breathing in. Your body is now filled with pure, healing air. Breathe this white light in and out for several minutes. When you are ready, open your eyes and get up slowly.

mini meditation
Avoiding temptation

If you feel like you want a cigarette or a drink, stop, relax your shoulders, and take a deep breath into your belly. As you breathe out, slowly let your shoulders drop further and say the words, 'I am clean and pure'. Repeat the exercise any time the desire creeps back to the front of your mind.

AVOIDING ENVIRONMENTAL HAZARDS

There is a wide range of situations and substances proven or suspected of being particularly toxic if trying to conceive or when pregnant. If you are aware of potential hazards, you should be able to take action against them. Learning to read labels is the first step.

Toxic substances are all around us – in our homes, gardens, and workplace; in some of the things we eat and drink; in many of the clothes we wear; and on the roads and streets we travel.

Toxic chemicals

Lead is present in exhaust fumes, petrol, paint and in some water. It can result in a low sperm count and a high number of abnormally shaped sperm and to reproductive problems in women.

To reduce your exposure, use unleaded petrol, drink filtered water and avoid driving on or walking near busy, polluted roads. Do not use paints and solder.

Mercury is used widely in dentistry, and in the production of pesticides and fungicides. It also is present in many fish. Mercury can decrease sperm production and have toxic effects on the ova. It also can cause birth defects in a developing fetus.

Have mercury fillings removed well before you plan to become pregnant and if you need a filling, make sure your dentists uses a non-mercury compound.

Avoid using weed killers and steer clear of public areas – parks, gardens, golf courses, and lawns – where they are certain to be used.

Cadmium is found in cigarettes, solder and some pesticides. It can cause poor sperm production and interfere with the implantation of a fertilised egg. Thus, you have another reason not to smoke or be around people who smoke!

Dioxins are a by-product of chlorine bleaching used in the production of toilet paper, sanitary towels, tea bags and milk cartons.

Cut down on your exposure by choosing non-chlorine-bleached paper products and buying milk in glass bottles.

Phosphates, chlorine, phenol and ammonia are found in many cleaners and disinfectants and are highly hazardous to reproduction.

Choose 'natural' products, where possible or make your own safe versions.

Phthalates These chemicals are found in many items used daily – cosmetics, cling film and other food packaging, fatty foods, house dust, PVC flooring and wiring, wallpaper and blinds, car seats, plasticized clothing; paints and adhesives.

Phthalates are not thought to be readily stored in the body because they have a short "half-life" (just 12 hours), yet tests on women show levels in urine remain constant. Some researchers put this down to daily use of cosmetics containing the chemicals (they are readily absorbed through skin). They may also be inhaled when they leach out of plastic.

Phthalates cross the placenta and are hormone-disrupting. Research links exposure to phthalates during pregnancy with changes in the way baby boys' genitals develop (including smaller penises and testicles not descending completely and premature breast development in girls.

Make sure you read all packaging carefully and choose more natural versions.

Solvents are widely used in industry and are known to have harmful effects on male and female reproductive systems. Chemicals as tetrachloroethylene and benzene are used in dry-cleaning fluids, hair and other dyes and paint strippers.

Make sure you read all labels carefully and avoid any products with these substances. If your work involves contact with strong chemicals, make sure you consult your doctor about any protective measures you can take to preserve fertility.

Artificial musks These are petrochemical-derived additives used to fragrance cosmetics, cleaning and laundry products. They adhere to clothing and accumulate in body fat after being absorbed through skin and food (the molecules pass from household wastewater into water sources, then fish and have been detected in breastmilk. Artificial musks are liver toxins linked with skin irritation.

Make sure you read all packaging carefully and choose more natural versions.

Biocides Added to products labelled antimicrobial and antibacterial, from handwashing liquid and toothpaste to paint for bathrooms and kitchens, these chemicals accumulate in the environment and may add to the development of drug-resistant superbugs.

Make sure you read all packaging carefully and choose more natural versions.

Radiation

Cosmic rays from the sky, radon as from the ground, power lines, mobile telephones, computers and microwaves all are sources of radiation and potentially damaging to the reproductive system and a developing fetus. If you live in a high-risk area for ionising radiation from radon gas, for example you need to take protective measures (contact the Environmental Protection Agency). You should avoid any unnecessary x-rays and limit non-essential air travel and consider reducing the amount of time you spend in front of the computer, talking on your mobile and microwaving.

Heat

Although not a problem for women, heat exposure can prove damaging to sperm so if your partner works in certain industries – bakeries, welding, firefighting, for example – or drives long distances, cycles in tight clothing or sits for long hours at his desk, he should take plenty of breaks outdoors, wear loose, cool clothing and have a cool shower after work.

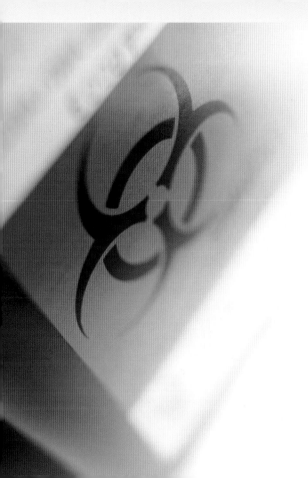

Lessening the effects of environmental hazards

✓ Use organic methods when gardening.
✓ Check out your water supply; replace any lead pipes and install a water filter..
✓ Buy organic food and eco cleaning materials.
✓ Try to schedule any necessary x-rays or dental treatment before you get pregnaunt.
✓ Consider having your house's radon levels checked.
✓ If your job involves working with chemicals – dry cleaner, dental nurse, hair colourist, for example; physical stress – nurse or manual worker; infection – nurse, vet, dentist or doctor, or travel – air steward or tour guide, have a risk assessment carried out to ensure you are protected.
✕ Do not undertake DIY projects that involve the use of chemical products – paint stripping, painting, pest proofing.

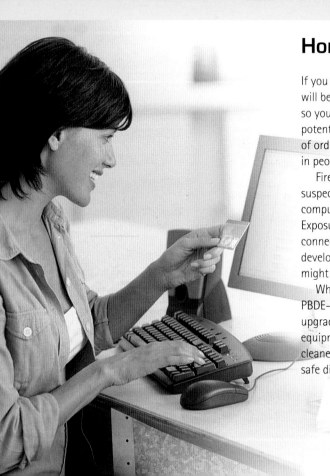

Home office hazards

If you work outside the home, your office or workspace will be monitored for safety and potential toxins. Not so your home workspace: a 2004 study by WWF found potentially hormone-disrupting chemicals in the blood of ordinary people at almost 10 times the levels found in people exposed through their occupations.

Fire-retardant chemicals or PBDEs that are suspected carcinogens have been detected in dust from computers of every make and age in many surveys. Exposure in the womb to these substances has been connected with a number of reproductive and developmental concerns. Moreover, a single monitor might comprise 2-4 kg lead.

When buying new electronic equipment ensure it's PBDE-free. Have a professional clean, repair and upgrade your PC in their own office and don't dump equipment irresponsibly. Vacuum with a HEPA-filter cleaner that traps dangerous dust and seals it in for safe disposal.

Garden hazards

Fertilizers, moss and weed killers, insecticides and rose products, slug and snail pellets all contain strong chemicals, some of which are neurotoxins. Watch out, too, for cleaners for tools, pots, kennels and hutches as they often contain reproductive and developmental toxins banned in the EU for domestic gardens.

Choose products marketed as 'eco garden' and throw out any existing products, especially if over a year old as they may contain newly banned substances.

Creosote is a particular danger. Banned for domestic use in 2003, old railway sleepers for bed edging may have been soaked in the stuff.

In 2004, the wood preservative used to treat over 90 percent of timber used for household decking, fences, picnic tables and children's play equipment was finally banned. It was made from the insecticide arsenic, a human carcinogen and reproductive toxin and was marketed as Wolmanised, tanalised, salt- or pressure-treated wood. In rain, arsenic washes from treated wood into soil and water sources.

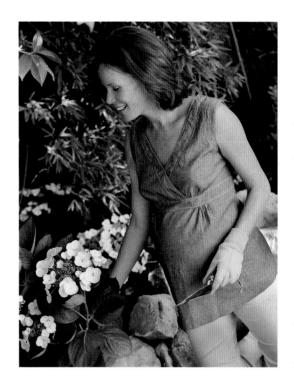

Celebrate your fertility

Use this meditation when you want to

- Regulate your menstrual cycle and return your body to a state of natural balance

- Relieve your anxieties about getting pregnant

- Increase your chances of conception

How to practise this meditation

This is an inspiring visualisation to perform outside if the weather is good. Sit comfortably, relax, close your eyes and focus on your breathing.

Now imagine that you are a seed, packed with the vital energy you need to grow into a wonderful fruit-bearing tree. You are planted in the earth, feeling safe, peaceful and nurtured. You are tranquil, yet eager to grow. Above you is a glimmer of sunlight and you feel an urge to grow towards it. As you start to stretch upwards you feel your energy begin to move and you push out roots to give you a firm foundation. Slowly you grow towards the sun, feeling it warming and welcoming you. Gentle raindrops refresh and nourish as you start to grow tall and strong. First leaves, then blossom appear on your branches, making you look and feel healthy and radiant. As a soft breeze causes the flower petals to fall to the ground, all your cares float off with them and you feel peaceful and happy. In place of the blossom, fruit begins to grow. It looks healthy, delicious and is growing bigger all the time.

Enjoy the pleasantly heavy sensation of this natural burden, congratulate yourself for having produced it and delight in the knowledge that you have achieved your purpose.

mini visualisation
Moments of doubt

If you are worrying about whether you will be able to get pregnant, try creating such a strong, positive image in your mind's eye that it pushes out any doubts or anxieties. Picture yourself, your partner and your beautiful baby together and happy in a special safe place. See the image so clearly that your brain accepts it as fact and tells your body to make it a reality.

HELP WITH CONCEPTION

The majority of couples will conceive within a year if they have sex two or three times a week. About seven out of ten couples will conceive within a month if they have sex every day, but only one or two couples will be successful if they have sex just once a week. Having sex infrequently increases the chances that you will be having intercourse at a time when you are not fertile, though having sex too frequently can lower a man's sperm count.

As well as frequency of intercourse, certain positions can make it easier for you to conceive (see page 64). More significant is if you are aware of your fertile times. Having sex at ovulation or on a few days either side of it is the critical time for conception.

Sperm can carry either an X (female) chromosome or a Y (male) chromosome. X-carrying sperm are thought to enjoy favourable conditions in the cervix in the days before ovulation and Y-carrying sperm benefit from conditions at ovulation or just after.

The easiest time for a woman to get pregnant is between the ages of 26 and 40. After the age of 40, only four or five out of every ten will conceive and only one in ten women over the age of 45 can expect to get pregnant within a year.

The effects of age on fit, healthy men are small, however, and many men remain fertile all their lives. Smoking and a lack of general fitness, however, will affect semen quality and thus a man's fertility.

An inability to conceive quickly is currently affecting about one in five couples and is expected to rise in the future. However, there are a number of techniques available to assist infertile couples. Current advice for couples under 35 having regular intercourse is not to seek treatment for infertility for at least a year unless a known problem exists. Older couples who have been trying to conceive without success for three to six months, should visit a doctor sooner.

Some facts about ova

- A woman is born with a life-time supply—approximately two million eggs, but they begin to die off from the moment of birth. By puberty, only about 400,000 will remain.
- Each month about 100 to 150 ova begin to ripen inside fluid-filled sacs called follicles; usually only one of these eggs reaches maturity.
- As soon as a single egg matures, oestrogen is released into the bloodstream stopping the ripening of other eggs.
- At ovulation, the egg is no more than a dot, barely visible to the human eye.
- The life span of an egg is up to five days.
- Ova contain only 'x' chromosomes.

Some facts about sperm

- Sperm development begins in puberty and continues throughout adulthood. The quantity and quality decrease from around age 40. Each sperm takes 72 days to develop.
- The average healthy young man produces 2-6ml of semen per ejaculation; each millilitre contains 50-150 million sperm.
- Each sperm measures 0.05mm in length.
- Only a few hundred sperm eventually arrive at the fallopian tubes; the fastest in about 45 minutes, the slowest in about 12 hours.
- The life span of a sperm is 12-24 hours.
- There are two types: male sperm that contain a 'y' chromosome and female sperm that contain an 'x' chromosome.

Sexual positions

There is an argument that any position that a couple enjoys and is comfortable performing is probably a good one for conception, though see the proviso below. While there is no evidence that remaining horizontal for 15 minutes or so after intercourse will allow more semen to remain in your vagina, it can't hurt to try. There are millions of sperm in every ejaculation, so there should be plenty of sperm in your vagina even if you get up right away.

However, if there is any chance that the woman has a retroverted uterus, one tilted backwards rather than forwards, than a man-on-top position will work well when trying to conceive. Placing a small pillow under the hips following intercourse so that the cervix rests in the pool of semen for a short time (perhaps 20 minutes or so) will expose the cervix to the greatest number of sperm and will allow the sperm time to easily swim up through the cervix. Or, with a tipped uterus, you may have better luck having intercourse from behind (hands and knees position), which allows the sperm better access to the cervix.

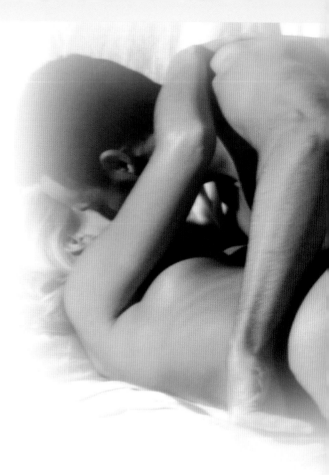

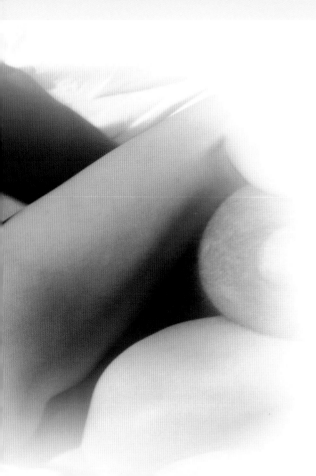

Positions to avoid

It makes sense for women to avoid straddling their partners while making love as this can cause more semen to leak out and may result in fewer sperm making their way to the egg. Therefore, woman-on-top, sitting or standing positions are not advisable if you want to conceive readily.

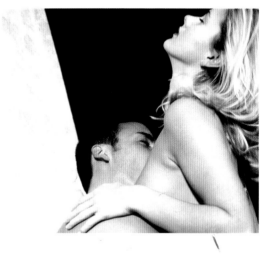

Recognising your fertile signs

During your menstrual cycle there are dozens of changes in your body, but two main ones can help you monitor your own fertility – the amount and consistency of your cervical mucus and the rise in basal body temperature (BBT). It's also possible to learn to recognise the changes in your cervix, breasts and overall mood that can signal ovulation.

Cervical mucus

The type of mucus secreted by your cervix is determined by the hormones oestrogen and progesterone. When oestrogen levels are high – just before ovulation – the mucus is profuse, clear, watery and stretchy. This is the most fertile form of mucus because it provides a nurturing alkaline medium for sperm, and encourages their speedy passage up the Fallopian tubes to the waiting ovum. The last day that you secrete fertile mucus is known as peak day. You are most fertile during the two or three days that you notice this clear, stretchy mucus leading up to, and including, peak day. When progesterone levels rise after ovulation, the mucus becomes thicker and then disappears. This thick mucus, however, forms an impenetrable plug, which may help to increase the chance of conception by keeping a reservoir of sperm in the cervical canal after ovulation. Because sperm have a life span of up to five days, this plug allows the maximum time for a sperm to fertilise the waiting ovum successfully.

BBT (Basal Body Temperature)

The normal human body temperature averages at about 37°C (98.6°F) but varies during the day, especially in response to exercise. A woman's body temperature also responds to hormonal changes throughout the month, and signals changes in fertility. The BBT is at its lowest level during the menstrual cycle and through to ovulation. Soon after ovulation, however, the BBT rises at least 0.2°C (approximately 0.4°F) and stays raised until menstruation starts; this is the second or post-ovulatory phase. The rise in temperature is due to the hormone progesterone, which is secreted by the corpus luteum after the ovum has been released, and is a sign that ovulation has already occurred.

Reading the signs

- Immediately after your period you will produce very little cervical mucus; probably you will feel dry around the vagina.
- A few more days into your cycle and you will begin to feel more slippery around your vagina; you may notice some sticky or creamy mucus.
- As ovulation nears, your mucus increases in quantity and becomes clear and stretchy. This is a sign of your fertility.
- If you have intercourse on any of the days that you secrete the slippery, clear and stretchy mucus, you could conceive. However, the most fertile day is usually when the mucus is at its clearest and stretchiest, although not always at its most profuse.

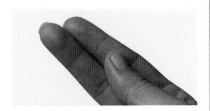

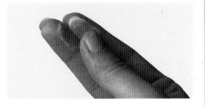

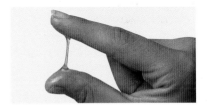

So that you can take your BBT accurately, you will need to purchase a special glass fertility thermometer, which has each degree marked in tenths or an unbreakable electronic digital thermometer. The latter makes a beeping sound when a stable temperature is reached and stores the information until you are ready to read or record it. If you are using a glass fertility thermometer remember to shake it down well first.

You can record your temperature from your mouth, vagina or rectum but be consistent: your BBT will be slightly different depending on which route you choose. If you use a glass thermometer, leave it in place for five minutes before reading the temperature. If the mercury falls between two numbers record the lowest temperature every time. A digital thermometer will need about a minute to "beep" with a reading.

A rise in your BBT confirms that your mucus is fertile. Because the temperature rise is caused by progesterone secreted by the corpus luteum after ovulation, it occurs too late to be used as a fertility signal; the ovum has deteriorated and cannot be fertilised. However, if you seem to be having problems getting pregnant, charting your temperature will help you identify possible causes, such as early or late ovulation, lack of ovulation altogether, or even very early miscarriage.

Bear in mind that every woman is different and you will need to learn your own unique set of monthly fertility signals.

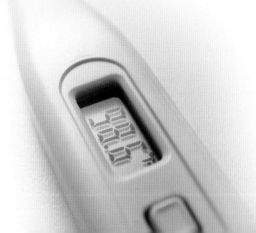

'High-tech' aids

There are a couple of devices that use the body's natural fertility signals and combine them with modern technology to help you predict your most fertile time. Although these give an accurate result when performed at the right time, they can be expensive and difficult to use if you have an irregular cycle.

Ovulation predictor kits

Most use urine to detect the surge of luteinising hormone (LH) that triggers ovulation. They are usually very accurate if the urine tests are performed at the right time, but you still need to keep a record of your periods to be able to calculate approximately when you should test for the LH surge.

A typical kit contains five urine-testing sticks, which need to be used on consecutive days around the time of ovulation. If you have a regular cycle, you can start testing about 17 days before you expect a period, but if your cycle is at all irregular you could easily miss the five-day fertility window. In this case, you could either buy several kits, or you could simply learn to read your cervical mucus (see page 77), perhaps using a test kit to confirm ovulation.

Saliva test kits also are available. These use the fact that saliva will mirror the changes in chervical mucus during the fertility cycle.

Computerised fertility predictor

This small monitor stores data from your previous menstrual cycles and your daily BBT to predict the days you are fertile. It can be used to indicate infertile times and if your BBT is persistently raised, as in the case of pregnancy. However, it gives a false sense of accuracy because the information it provides is based on previous cycles until your BBT rises, which signals the start of your infertile phase.

Other fertility signals

Sometimes a woman may feel a sharp pain or dull ache low down and to one side of her abdomen when she ovulates. The medical term for this mid-cycle pain is *mittelschmerz*, which is German for 'middle pain'. It may be a momentary twinge or can last for 24 hours and be quite uncomfortable. Studies using ultrasound scans to see what happens when a woman ovulates show that this symptom does not always coincide precisely with ovulation and can be felt just before or after the ovum is released.

A tiny loss of blood sometimes occurs around the time of ovulation, but if you notice this you should see your doctor to check that your cervix is healthy before putting the bleeding down to ovulation as it could be a sign of something that needs medical attention. You also may notice that your libido increases around the time of ovulation and decreases again in the infertile days leading up to your period.

Some women become aware that before their periods their breasts become more tender, slightly larger and feel denser or even lumpy. This is due to the progesterone circulating in the body after ovulation.

Occasionally, a woman can detect a small lymph node in her groin that swells when she ovulates. You can test yourself for this lymph node by feeling in your groin during the days when your fertile mucus appears: you may notice a pea-like swelling on one side. Remember, however, that lymph nodes or glands may also swell in this region for many other reasons, for instance, if you have a vaginal infection or flu.

Many women also experience premenstrual changes in mood but these may diminish as you begin to improve your health for pregnancy.

Using fertility awareness to conceive

Being aware of your fertile times can help you to conceive. The most important sign to look for is the slippery, clear and stretchy mucus. If you have intercourse on any of the days that you secrete this mucus you could conceive. However, the most fertile day is usually when the mucus is at its clearest and stretchiest, although not always at its most profuse. If you examine your cervix as well, you will be able to feel as it softens and opens up during your fertile phase.

To optimise your chances of conceiving, you should have intercourse when you notice a wet feeling or the slippery, clear mucus. Even if you have not yet ovulated, fertile mucus is designed to transport sperm towards the site of fertilisation and nurture them for up to five days, until an ovum is released. Try to have intercourse on the most fertile or peak day. This is usually the last day you notice fertile mucus and it should soon be followed by the temperature rise which confirms ovulation. Intercourse on one of the five days leading up to the temperature rise is most likely to result in pregnancy.

As fertile mucus helps to nurture and transport sperm, you don't need to have intercourse every day. In fact, having intercourse on alternate days once your cervical mucus appears should not only be sufficient, it may actually help to ensure a higher concentration of sperm in the semen than more frequent intercourse.

If you don't conceive immediately, don't worry. On average, only one in four fertile couples will conceive in a given month, despite having had intercourse at the 'right' time. It may take a few cycles for you to become familiar with your body's natural fertility signs, but once you do, you will have a much better idea of when is the right time to conceive. Just remember the three golden rules below about the days to have intercourse:

Have intercourse when your:
- Cervical mucus is fertile (clear and stretchy);
- Basal body temperature has not yet risen;
- Cervix is high, soft, open and central in the vagina.

FERTILITY TREATMENTS

In the early stages of trying for a baby, there are a number of complementary approaches you can try. These tend to be less invasive and cheaper than conventional fertility treatments. If, however, these are not appropriate, you will have to consider what assisted reproductive technology has to offer.

Having fertility treatment can leave you anticipating every treatment and awaiting test results in a state of almost permanent anxiety. It also can make you feel stressed and unhappy in your relationship or as if your life is on hold. Often, the best way to deal with fertility problems and increase your chances of conception is to take your mind off them completely. Rather than long for happiness in the future, just focus on how wonderful and blessed you can feel right at this moment. Try to do activities as a couple, including meditating together, and spend time with friends and allow yourself treats such as a romantic weekend away.

Becoming mindful of everyday events also can be therapeutic. Being engrossed in a task anchors you in the present, blots out anxieties and enables you to take pleasure in your life right now.

Complementary methods

Some couples who have problems conceiving are able to reverse the situation by changing their diet and lifestyle. If one of the partners has a nutritional deficiency or a body overloaded with toxins, fertility can be affected. In such cases, embarking on a 'conception' diet filled with essential nutrients can make all the difference. The first step is to have a vitamin and mineral assessment done.

Reflexology, acupuncture, herbal medicine and hypnotherapy are claimed to benefit fertility and if one of these appeals to you, then you need to consult a qualified practitioner.

ART (assisted reproductive technology)

Techniques available include ovulation induction, intrauterine insemination, in vitro fertilisation and the micro-manipulation techniques of intracytoplasmic sperm injection and assisted hatching. Your doctor will determine the method(s) that will be the best for you and your partner depending on your medical histories, any underlying reproductive problems and more personal factors such as time and cost.

OI (ovulation induction)

About 30 percent of infertile women have ovulation disorders and certain 'fertility drugs', may help them achieve ovulation. The drugs are inexpensive and can be taken over a three- to six-month period. If pregnancy does not occur during this time, ovulation induction is unlikely to result in pregnancy and other types of treatment will be needed to conceive.

Common reasons for infertility

Woman

There are three main reasons why a woman may not be able to conceive:
- Failure to ovulate;
- Failure of the ovum to unite with a sperm (caused, for example, by blocked fallopian tubes or hostile cervical mucus);
- Inability to sustain a growing fetus.

Man

Infertility in the male is limited to problems with sperm including:
- Failure to produce sufficient healthy sperm, including both a lack of sperm or the production of poor-quality sperm;
- Inability to deliver the sperm into the vagina due both to a physical problem or emotional difficulties.

IVF (in vitro fertilisation)

The most popular method of assisted conception, this involves fertilising a woman's eggs outside her body under controlled laboratory conditions and replacing the resulting embryos back into her uterus. A couple can use their own eggs and sperm, frozen embryos, or egg and sperm donated from anonymous donors. Typically, fresh embryos are used in the first treatment cycle, while the remaining embryos may be frozen and used in subsequent treatments.

IVF has been successful for women with irreparable fallopian tube damage, endometriosis, ovulatory disorders; for men with sub-optimal sperm and for couples with unexplained infertility. Success rates do vary widely but the average is 25–30 per cent.

IUI (intrauterine or 'artificial' insemination)

Less invasive and expensive than other methods of assisted conception for many couples, in this procedure, sperm is inserted directly into a woman's uterus at the time of ovulation to meet an ovum and fertilise it.

If you've been trying to conceive for quite some time and are considering what to do next, you should consider intrauterine insemination. If you decide to have IUI, you will be offered the option of using the woman's natural cycle in which only one egg is released, or increasing the number of eggs released by using fertility drugs. The latter tends to have higher success rates.

IUI can help to improve the chances of conception for couples with unexplained infertility, women with endometriosis and men with mildly reduced sperm quality. Success rates for IUI are between 10-15 per cent per cycle depending on the age of the woman, the quality of the sperm and how long the couple have been infertile.

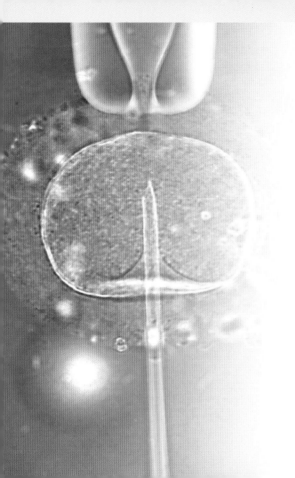

ICSI (intracytoplasmic sperm injection)

If the man has sub-optimal sperm, ICSI can greatly improve a couple's chance of pregnancy. In this technique, sperm is injected directly into the zona pellucida (the 'egg shell') of the ovum. The majority of infertile males produce sperm, which are unable to pentrate the ovum's outer coating. Microinjection of sperm directly into an egg has been successful since 1991. Over 90 per cent of couples treated by ICSI achieve fertilisation; the fertilisation rate per egg is about 60 per cent.

AH (assisted hatching)

This technique improves the implantation of any embryos. The zona pellucida ('egg shell') is breached to allow the embryo to break free (hatch) and implant into the uterine lining. This technique may be helpful in women over 40 years of age. Women undergoing this procedure are required to take special drugs (antibiotics and steroids).

Make the most of fertility treatments

Use this meditation when you want to	How to practise this meditation

• Trust in your ability to conceive
 	
• Make a decision about whether or not to embark on fertility treatment
 	
• Take more pleasure in the present
 	
• Find the resources to cope with stressful procedures
	Begin by sitting comfortably and focus on your breathing. Just be aware of the movement of your breath and the way it enters and leaves your body. Worries, anxieties, hopes and dreams will continue to flood your mind so just sit quietly and watch each thought come and go.
	
	    Be aware of how your thought process works, how different ideas keep appearing and disappearing and vying for attention. Observe the process but try not to get carried along with the thoughts; if you do, just return to observing your breath and how it is moving at this moment in your body.
	
	    Do not be too hard on yourself if you do lose concentration, however, just accept that it happens, let

your thoughts go, and return to your breath and the present. As you end your meditation know that at any time you can let go of your worries about the future and just be relaxed in the present.

mini visualisation
During treatments

At times of particular stress, anxiety, fear or pain, you can remain calm by practising a mini meditation. Just find an object of interest in the car, waiting room or clinic where you are being treated and focus on it to the exclusion of all else. It could be a plant, a picture or the view through a window. Don't stare at it, just relax, half close your eyes, let your breathing find a slow, natural rhythm and explore the object in such detail that there is no room for anxieties to nudge their way in.

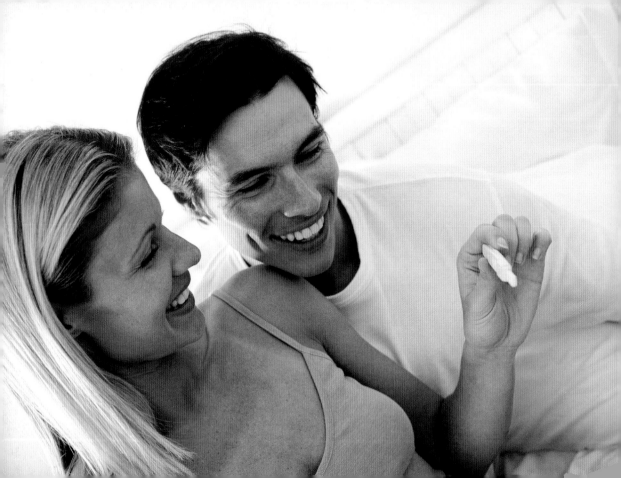

Chapter 2

The first trimester

JUST PREGNANT

The first twelve weeks of your pregnancy, known as the first trimester, can be among the most thrilling in your life. Although your body may not look different, you are almost certain to feel different – both physically and emotionally – thanks to the enormous changes taking place inside you. These first three months are the most significant in terms of fetal development, so it is particularly important to nurture yourself and your baby during these crucial early weeks.

Whether this is your first child or your third, the excitement of discovering that you have created and are nurturing a new life is a truly wonderful experience. Some women sail through pregnancy without giving much thought to what is happening inside them. And yet there is more than just a tiny embryo developing, day-by-day, inside the uterus: pregnancy represents the beginning of the growth of a unique individual. It also signifies the start of a new phase in your life and that of your partner.

Pregnancy signs

While some women just intuitively know they've become pregnant, you don't have to 'feel' pregnant to actually be pregnant. There are certain telltale symptoms of pregnancy, and while you might experience all, it's more likely that you'll only be affected by a few.

Missing a period

This is one of the clearest indications of pregnancy. However, stress, illness, extreme fluctuations in weight – excessive gain or anorexia – or coming off the oral contraceptive pill can all stop periods for a while. Irregular periods are a common symptom with polycystic ovary syndrome, a condition in which periods can occur several months apart.

Breast tenderness

Changes in the size and feel of your breasts will occur just a few days after conception; your breasts will begin to enlarge in readiness for breastfeeding, and you'll probably experience heaviness and soreness. Many women report that their breasts are very sensitive and experience a sharp, tingling sensation, too.

Nausea and vomiting

Feeling sick is the most common complaint in early pregnancy. Most women are affected from around five to six weeks of pregnancy, but some may be nauseated as early as two weeks after conception. Although termed 'morning sickness', the nausea can occur at any

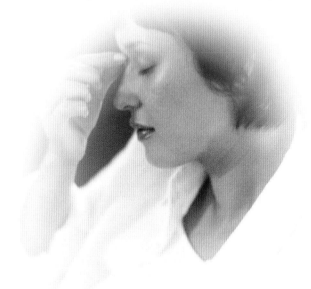

time of day and can vary from an occasional, faint sensation to an overwhelming feeling of nausea and vomiting. By and large, these symptoms disappear by around 14 to 16 weeks of pregnancy.

Tiredness

Many women report feelings of extreme tiredness during early pregnancy. Typically, after getting in from work in the evening, all you want to do is go to bed, or you may be desperate for a mid-afternoon nap. When you reach week 14 of your pregnancy, your energy levels should start to pick up.

Frequent urination

As early as two weeks after conception. you will find yourself wanting to urinate more frequently due to the pressure of the enlarging uterus on the bladder. At about 14 weeks, the uterus rises up into the abdomen, which often relieves this annoying symptom until the last few weeks of pregnancy when the baby's head engages (drops down in the uterus), again causing pressure on your bladder. Rising levels of progesterone

also stimulate the bladder muscle so that you feel your bladder is full even when there's not much urine in there. In addition to this, your kidneys are working harder in response to being pregnant, and an extra 6 to 7 litres (13 to 15 pts) will be added to your circulation to increase the blood flow around your body.

Changes in taste and smell

Certain foods may suddenly make you feel queasy or you may start to crave particular foods or even certain smells. You also may have a strange metallic taste in your mouth.

Constipation

A common early symptom of pregnancy, this is caused by high levels of progesterone, which relaxes the bowel and slows your digestion

Mood swings

High levels of pregnancy hormones flood your body in early pregnancy, making you extra emotional and sometimes weepy.

Pregnancy tests

Two weeks after conception your baby is just a ball of cells, not much bigger than a pinhead, starting to develop in the lining of the uterus. Already the placenta is forming and starting to produce a hormone called human chorionic gonadotrophin (HCG), which passes into your bloodstream and urine from the day of your first missed period and which can be detected by special pregnancy tests.

Home pregnancy tests

Available from most chemists, these are very accurate and can be performed from the first day that you've missed your period. There are several different home kits on the market, so always read the manufacturer's instructions carefully.

You should use the first urine passed when you get up as this is the most concentrated; urine passed later in the day will be diluted by what you drink and eat, so very early pregnancy hormone levels may be too low for a home kit to detect.

Some tests ask you to hold a stick in your urine flow, others require that you pass urine into a clean

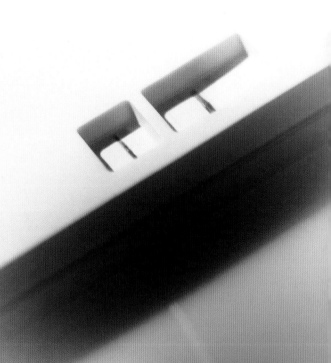

container and then use a dropper to squeeze a few drops onto a window on an oblong stick.

Usually the result appears within minutes and can be read by looking for a coloured line in a window on the stick. Often there is also a line indicating that the test has been carried out correctly. If the test is negative, but you still feel that you may be pregnant, repeat the test in five to seven days. It may be that the pregnancy is too early to detect and you became pregnant later than you thought. This is most likely if you have irregular periods.

Internal examination

Four to six weeks after conception, telltale signs such as the uterus softening and an alteration in the texture of the cervix will be discernible on an internal examination. The vaginal tissues thicken and produce more secretions, resulting in a heavier discharge. The uterus grows so quickly – it's already about the size of a small orange by eight weeks – that its size can help your doctor to date a pregnancy accurately. However, in practice, if you are sure of your dates and your pregnancy test is positive, your doctor will not need to examine you internally.

Pregnancy blood tests

If urine tests are inconclusive, your healthcare provider may use a blood test to detect and date a pregnancy. The test may simply give you a positive or negative result, or it may test levels of HCG, depending on your symptoms and medical history. The more sophisticated blood tests can detect a pregnancy from as early as two weeks after conception. Pregnancy blood tests are useful if there are any concerns about miscarriage or if your healthcare provider suspects an ectopic pregnancy. In these situations HCG blood levels don't usually rise as fast and may even fall, indicating that the pregnancy has failed.

Calculating your delivery date

Once your pregnancy's been confirmed, one of the first things you'll want to know is when your baby will be born. Your pregnancy is dated from the first day of your last menstrual period (LMP). If you have a regular 28-day cycle and know the date of the first day of your LMP, you can count on nine months plus seven days – or 280 days – after the first day of your LMP. You can adjust the date according to the length of your cycle. If you have a 26-day cycle, count on nine months plus five days from your LMP – or 278 days. If you have a 32-day cycle, count on nine months plus 11 days from your LMP – or 284 days – and so on.

Alternatively, use the chart opposite. Locate the date that your last menstrual period began by looking at the months and numbers in bold. Then look at the number (and month) directly below it; this represents your EDD. If, for instance, your LMP was on 12 April, your baby will be due on 17 January the following year. Remember, however, that this is just a general guide – only about 5 per cent of babies are born on their estimated birth dates.

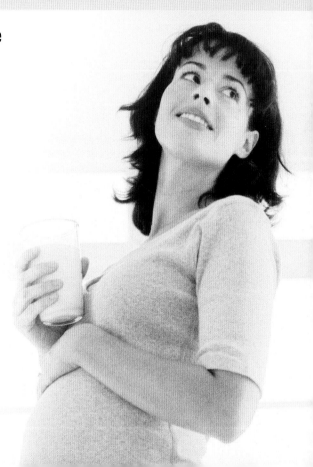

	1	2	3	4	5	6	7	8	9	10	11	12	13	14	15	16	17	18	19	20	21	22	23	24	25	26	27	28	29	30	31
January	1	2	3	4	5	6	7	8	9	10	11	12	13	14	15	16	17	18	19	20	21	22	23	24	25	26	27	28	29	30	31
Oct/Nov	8	9	10	11	12	13	14	15	16	17	18	19	20	21	22	23	24	25	26	27	28	29	30	31	1	2	3	4	5	6	7
February	1	2	3	4	5	6	7	8	9	10	11	12	13	14	15	16	17	18	19	20	21	22	23	24	25	26	27	28			
Nov/Dec	8	9	10	11	12	13	14	15	16	17	18	19	20	21	22	23	24	25	26	27	28	29	30	1	2	3	4	5			
March	1	2	3	4	5	6	7	8	9	10	11	12	13	14	15	16	17	18	19	20	21	22	23	24	25	26	27	28	29	30	31
Dec/Jan	6	7	8	9	10	11	12	13	14	15	16	17	18	19	20	21	22	23	24	25	26	27	28	29	30	31	1	2	3	4	5
April	1	2	3	4	5	6	7	8	9	10	11	12	13	14	15	16	17	18	19	20	21	22	23	24	25	26	27	28	29	30	
Jan/Feb	6	7	8	9	10	11	12	13	14	15	16	17	18	19	20	21	22	23	24	25	26	27	28	29	30	31	1	2	3	4	
May	1	2	3	4	5	6	7	8	9	10	11	12	13	14	15	16	17	18	19	20	21	22	23	24	25	26	27	28	29	30	31
Feb/Mar	5	6	7	8	9	10	11	12	13	14	15	16	17	18	19	20	21	22	23	24	25	26	27	28	1	2	3	4	5	6	7
June	1	2	3	4	5	6	7	8	9	10	11	12	13	14	15	16	17	18	19	20	21	22	23	24	25	26	27	28	29	30	
Mar/Apr	8	9	10	11	12	13	14	15	16	17	18	19	20	21	22	23	24	25	26	27	28	29	30	31	1	2	3	4	5	6	
July	1	2	3	4	5	6	7	8	9	10	11	12	13	14	15	16	17	18	19	20	21	22	23	24	25	26	27	28	29	30	31
Apr/May	7	8	9	10	11	12	13	14	15	16	17	18	19	20	21	22	23	24	25	26	27	28	29	30	1	2	3	4	5	6	7
August	1	2	3	4	5	6	7	8	9	10	11	12	13	14	15	16	17	18	19	20	21	22	23	24	25	26	27	28	29	30	31
May/Jun	8	9	10	11	12	13	14	15	16	17	18	19	20	21	22	23	24	25	26	27	28	29	30	31	1	2	3	4	5	6	7
September	1	2	3	4	5	6	7	8	9	10	11	12	13	14	15	16	17	18	19	20	21	22	23	24	25	26	27	28	29	30	
Jun/Jul	8	9	10	11	12	13	14	15	16	17	18	19	20	21	22	23	24	25	26	27	28	29	30	1	2	3	4	5	6	7	
October	1	2	3	4	5	6	7	8	9	10	11	12	13	14	15	16	17	18	19	20	21	22	23	24	25	26	27	28	29	30	31
Jul/Aug	8	9	10	11	12	13	14	15	16	17	18	19	20	21	22	23	24	25	26	27	28	29	30	31	1	2	3	4	5	6	7
November	1	2	3	4	5	6	7	8	9	10	11	12	13	14	15	16	17	18	19	20	21	22	23	24	25	26	27	28	29	30	
Aug/Sept	8	9	10	11	12	13	14	15	16	17	18	19	20	21	22	23	24	25	26	27	28	29	30	31	1	2	3	4	5	6	
December	1	2	3	4	5	6	7	8	9	10	11	12	13	14	15	16	17	18	19	20	21	22	23	24	25	26	27	28	29	30	31
Sept/Oct	7	8	9	10	11	12	13	14	15	16	17	18	19	20	21	22	23	24	25	26	27	28	29	30	1	2	3	4	5	6	7

Welcome the new life inside you

Use this meditation when you want to

- Celebrate the creation of a new life

- Start bonding with your child

- Accept you're pregnant even if there are no visible signs

How to practise this meditation

Find a place that is quiet and comfortable. Assume a comfortable position that you can hold without difficulty for the duration of the meditation.

Start by gently shaking out the tensions in your muscles and then ease yourself into a lying position. Once you feel settled, concentrate on your breathing until it is slow and calm. Now divide your body into seven distinct sections: scalp and forehead; face and neck; shoulders, arms and hands; chest and back; diaphragm and solar plexus; belly; and hips, legs and feet. This will allow you to focus intimately on each one in turn.

Beginning at the top of your head and working slowly down to the tips of your toes, concentrate all

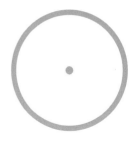

your attention on each section for the duration of a few breaths, clenching the muscles in each part of your body on the inhalation and releasing the tension as you breathe out. Focus on the flow of your breathing, especially in and out of your abdomen, and be aware of the sensations in your breasts and belly. This will make you more aware of the subtle changes that are taking place in your body.

With a visual aid

To give yourself a more concrete focus, you could use a visual aid. Draw a circle with a dot in the middle to represent life and its eternity. Now, without analysing the circle or its meaning, let your eyes move over the image, and familiarise yourself with it. Try shutting your eyes and keeping the image of the circle in your mind. Continue to be aware of your breathing but don't count your breaths as this shifts your focus of attention. Accept any thoughts that arise, but just let them float away, concentrating only on the circle. Remain aware of the physical sensations of the meditation as you focus on the circle, so that your baby's presence becomes linked with the way you feel in your body.

The meditation should last approximately fifteen minutes. The first few times you try this you could set a timer to let you know when it is time gently to open your eyes and come out of the meditation.

HEALTHY EATING

The first twelve weeks are the most important in your baby's development: the heart forms between the third and sixth weeks in utero, the buds that will develop into the limbs begin forming between the fourth and seventh weeks, and by the end of the first trimester, your child's basic brain structure and a rudimentary nervous system also will be in place.

In order to thrive during this crucial time, your baby needs to grow in his own small sanctuary. And in many ways the preservation of that sanctuary is in your hands. It is important to avoid stressful situations, to abstain from harmful substances such as alcohol and nicotine (see page 00), and to nurture your child by eating a balanced diet.

There's no great mystery to eating well in pregnancy; you simply need to eat a diet that's balanced in terms of the different food groups and contains sufficient nutrients. Analyze what you eat each day using the information on page 49, and you'll probably discover that you're already following a fairly healthy diet.

Pregnancy isn't a time for radical change, so don't switch from being a meat-eater to a vegetarian or vice versa; it can take your body months to adjust to such a drastic difference in diet. It's much better to adapt your current eating habits so your baby receives the best nourishment possible. If you're concerned that you're not eating enough from a particular food group, speak to your healthcare provider or a dietician, who will be able to advise you on your individual requirements.

Calorie needs

You'd assume that with a baby on the way, you'd need to eat twice as much food. In fact, you only need to eat about 2000 calories daily until your last trimester. However, requirements do vary with individual circumstances, and if you're concerned about your weight, speak to your healthcare provider.

If you were underweight when you started your pregnancy, are expecting twins or triplets, or are a teenager, you'll need more calories. If you're overweight, you'll probably be advised to keep your weight gain to a minimum until the last trimester.

Expecting twins

Although there are no specific guidelines in the UK for nutrition for twin or multiple pregnancies, it is generally accepted that there is a need for additional calories and nutrients throughout their pregnancy.

In fact gaining adequate weight in the first 20 weeks predicts a higher birth weight for the babies. The US Institute of Medicine recommends that regardless of pre-pregnancy weight, women pregnant with twins need to gain between 16-20 kg (35-45 lbs). Some of this – say 2.5 kg (5 lb) – should be in the first trimester.

Women expecting triplets may need to gain a total of around 23 kg (50 lb), or 0.7 kg (1.5 lb) per week.

To support the additional increases in blood volume and size of uterus as well as the development of more than one baby, more calcium, essential fatty acids and iron are needed, Your diet should contain a good mix of nurient rich foods and probably a good all-round antenatal supplement, particularly in the second trimester.

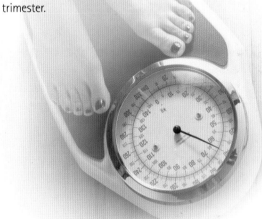

Food cravings and aversions

Developing a passion for certain foods is very common, particularly in early pregnancy. Spicy or pickled items, sweets and chocolate, milk, fruit and fruit juices and very cold foods like ice cream, are the most common cravings. On the other hand, you may develop a sudden aversion to some foods like meat or tea or coffee. In general, as long as your cravings or aversions don't prevent you from following a sensible diet most of the time, indulge yourself and don't worry. If you find, however, that you're missing out on a food that's a valuable source of nutrients, try to make up for any lack by substituting it for a food of similar nutritional value from the same food group (see page 49).

Fluids

An adequate fluid intake is essential during pregnancy, to help your blood volume increase and supply your baby with nutrients and because pregnancy raises your body temperature, to prevent dehydration. Aim to drink at least eight 225-ml (8-oz) glasses of water every day. However, milk, herbal teas and fruit and vegetable juices also are good choices.

In fact, during the first trimester when you may not feel like eating very much due to nausea, a fruit or vegetable smoothie can supply needed nutrients or ginger tea can help ease the nausea symptoms.

Limit your intake of caffeinated drinks (see page 52), as they can dehydrate you and have a deleterious effect on your baby. The current Food Standards Agency recommendation of a safe upper limit for pregnant women is 200 mg of caffeine per day.

Alcohol

You wouldn't be alone if you go off alcohol in pregnancy, and this is perhaps one of nature's ways of indicating that it is best avoided. Alcohol can restrict the amount of nutrients your baby obtains, both by limiting your appetite and by interfering with the function of the placenta. Regularly drinking two or more units of alcohol a day (see below for examples of a single unit) and binge drinking can cause miscarriage, low birth weight and permanent damage to your baby including mental, emotional, cognitive, social and behavioural difficulties, as well as physical deformities.

With all these possible effects, health professionals with an in-depth knowledge of fetal alcohol syndrome state that it is best to drink no alcohol at all while pregnant. Your doctor may tell you consuming one or two small glasses of wine a week with food does not seem to have any harmful effects but the reality is that there is no established safe limit for alcohol consumption in pregnancy and individuals can have differing levels of alcohol tolerance. The safest advice is to avoid alcohol throughout pregnancy. No drink = no risk!

Half a pint of beer
(284 ml or 10 fl oz)

A glass of wine
(85 ml or 3 fl oz)

An aperitif
(50 ml or 2 fl oz)

A measure of spirits
(25 ml or ¾ fl oz)

1st trimester needs

If you were consuming ideal levels of all vitamins before you were pregnant (see page 56), then, providing you eat the same diet, this will generally provide your baby with sufficient except for folate, one of the B group vitamins.

Unlike most vitamins, minerals are not 'manufactured' by the body and need to be consumed in food. Iron, calcium and zinc are particularly important during pregnancy and, you should also make sure that you get an adequate intake of iodine, magnesium and selenium, which are involved in a range of functions, from the regulation of your metabolism to the development of genetic material.

Folates and folic acid

Studies have shown that women can reduce drastically the risk of giving birth to a baby with a neural tube defect such as spina bifida by taking a folic acid supplement before conception and during the first 12 weeks, at which time the baby's neural tube has formed completely and the vulnerable period has passed.

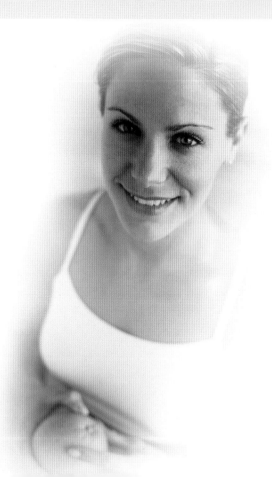

Folates are found naturally in foods such as green leafy vegetables, oranges and bananas but these alone are unlikely to provide adequate amounts so it's advisable to take a 400 mcg folic acid supplement and to eat foods fortified with folic acid, such as bread and breakfast cereals.

In contrast to other vitamins, folic acid (the synthetic version of the vitamin) is more readily absorbed than the natural version.

Vitamin A

Found in two forms – retinol in animal foods and beta carotene in plant foods – both a chronic lack or a high dose of retinol can cause fetal malformations, so getting the balance right is important. It is needed throughout your pregnancy for your baby's cell growth, and is vital in the first trimester for the development of your baby's heart and circulatory and nervous systems. It also helps to keep your skin and the linings of your internal organs healthy. Good sources of beta carotene are sweet potatoes, carrots, squash, spinach and mangoes while reduced-fat dairy products such as milk, yogurt, fromage frais and cheese, should be consumed for their retinol content.

Selenium

This antioxidant is essential for protecting cells against damage and a deficiency has been linked with miscarriage. Good sources include Brazil nuts, red meats, fish and selenium-enriched bread.

Magnesium

Along with calcium this is also important for proper bone growth. A recent study found that the amount of magnesium consumed in the first trimester was related to the weight, length and head circumference of your baby at birth.

Magnesium is essential for all muscle health, including your uterus. It also helps to make and repair tissue. Luckily, it is plentiful in salad greens, nuts, soya beans, seeds (particularly pumpkin, melon and sunflower) and whole grains.

Vegetarians and vegans

It is important if you are eating a meatless diet to eat a wide range of different foods from the main food groups in order to be supplied with key nutrients. Of particular concern for vegetarians is getting sufficient protein, iron, calcium, zinc and vitamins D and B12.

It is important not to rely solely on protein-rich dairy foods or eggs for protein, but to include beans, peas and lentils with grains in the diet. Soya products

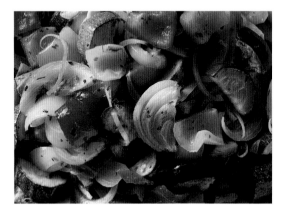

and beans are high in protein and also contain calcium and, if fortified, other vitamins and minerals such as essential B vitamins and iron. They also provide fibre. Nuts and seeds, such as sunflower and pumpkin, also provide useful nutrients.

During pregnancy your blood volume increases by 1.7 litres (3 pints) and iron is a key component of red blood cells. Many women, vegetarian or not, are prescribed iron supplements, but you should try to eat iron-rich foods, too. Good sources include lentils, beans, fortified cereals, eggs, dark green leafy vegetables, tofu, wholemeal bread and dried fruits. Avoid having tea or coffee with your meals to prevent the polyphenols that these drinks contain interfering with iron absorption. Instead, drink a glass of vitamin C-rich unsweetened fruit juice with your meals to increase iron absorption.

For vegetarians, getting vitamin D can be a problem, as oily fish, butter and margarines are the main dietary sources. A daily supplement of 10 micrograms a day is recommended for all pregnant women.

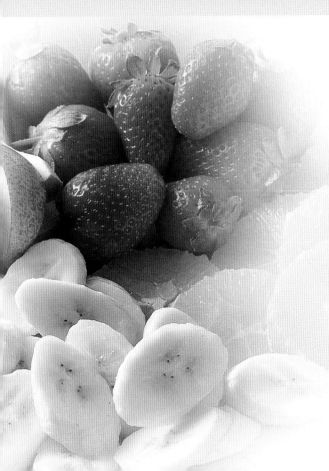

If you are an ovo-lacto vegetarian, calcium can easily be supplied by milk and dairy products, so have at least half a pint of milk a day, plus yogurt, fromage frais or cheese. Also try vegan sources such as white bread, tofu, chickpeas, almonds and fortified soya drinks.

Zinc is found in seeds cereals, brown rice and pasta and is plentiful in cheese and eggs.

If you are vegan, you must be particularly vigilant about your diet, and may be advised to consider having supplements or including a few animal products. Vegans tend to have lower birth weight babies and so it is crucial to eat properly, making sure you have sufficient calories and nutrients. Vitamin B12 is the one vitamin vegans really need to be concerned about. A supplement of B12 (combined with folic acid as they work together) is recommended.

Encourage your baby's healthy development

Use this meditation when you want to

- Find the strength to give up things that are not good for your baby

- Banish worries about a particular aspect of your pregnancy

- Relax your mind and body, which will benefit your baby

How to practise this meditation

Choose some place, perhaps in the garden if you have one or a quiet spot in the park, where you can see or hear signs of nature to give you a sense of the life growing within you. If you are new to meditating, you may find being outside too distracting when you are trying to focus. If this is the case, try sitting instead in the room that you have chosen as your sanctuary; this will have a calming influence that helps you focus. You may like to have a vase of fragrant flowers with you as you meditate.

Once you are comfortable, close your eyes and focus on the rhythm of your breathing by counting each in-breath. Concentrate on the changes in your body as you inhale and exhale. Think of your breaths as the unseen but very real presence of your baby – you cannot see it, but you know it is there every minute of the day. When your breathing has become balanced and regular, start using it to complement an affirmation. Choose one of the affirmations below, or alternatively use one of your own. Let the knowledge that each breath is carrying oxygen to your baby support the positive message of the affirmation. Practise repeating the phrase until it's instantly soothing; you can also use it as a mini meditation when you're out and about, to calm any nagging fears as they arise.

Using an affirmation creates a mental and physical state that not only encourages your child's healthy development but also calms you down and counteracts any negative thoughts that cross your mind. It's a way of confirming that you want the best for your baby and of blocking any distracting thoughts. It should pervade your mind until it's no longer just a collection of words but a part of you.

- I am the carrier of a healthy growing baby
- My body is a safe haven for my baby
- My baby is safe and well within me
- My baby is a unique human being

EXERCISE

Pregnancy makes demands on both your mind and your body. Exercising and using relaxation techniques can help you to maintain your health and sense of wellbeing. Physical activity causes the brain to release serotonin, dopamine and endorphins, chemicals, which help to balance mood swings, reduce stress and promote a positive outlook. At a time when your body is changing dramatically, exercising can give you a much-needed sense of control over your body image.

It will improve your heart and lung fitness and your posture, boost your circulation, help to control excessive weight gain, reduce digestive discomfort, relieve muscle aches and cramp and strengthen muscles. Working out in pregnancy may carry certain risks, so check with your healthcare provider before you begin or continue with an existing exercise programme.

If you haven't previously done much exercise, seek advice before embarking upon an exercise programme. You may be advised against starting a new regime until your second trimester, when the risk of miscarriage and overheating has decreased, and you're likely to have more energy. Bear in mind, too, that pregnancy is a time to maintain, rather than improve, fitness, and you should never work out with the intention of losing weight.

Relaxation

It is also important to spend time relaxing (see page 226) and not overly taxing yourself. Constantly rushing and trying to fit too many things into one day is the quickest way to exhaustion. Frenetic action not only increases your metabolic rate and stress levels, it also wastes precious energy. Try the meditation on page 116, when you feel you've too much on your plate.

Dos and don'ts of exercise

Pregnancy isn't a time to push yourself. Try to avoid or limit any strenuous activities, and always go at your own pace. Rest frequently, and take care not to overdo it, particularly in the first trimester. Always err on the side of caution – if you're in doubt about an exercise, don't do it.

You'll feel more motivated and are more likely to keep active if you enjoy what you do. However, do not engage in activities in which you're in danger of falling, losing your balance or getting hit in the stomach, such as horseback riding, roller blading, downhill skiing or team sports such as basketball or volleyball. Avoid scuba diving throughout pregnancy; it can cause gas bubbles to form in your baby's bloodstream.

At altitudes greater than 2500 metres take particular care not to overexert yourself and spend four to five days acclimitising. Check your heart rate to gauge how hard you're working.

When exercising, try to keep your breathing even and regular. Don't hold your breath at any point, as this increases pressure in your chest and can make you feel dizzy or faint.

Do not exercise if you

✕ Experience more than 6-8 uterine contractions per hour, a reduction in fetal movement or spotting or bleeding.

✕ Have a history of recurrent miscarriage or premature labour in previous pregnancies.

✕ Suffer from anaemia, respiratory disorders or cardiovascular disease, such as high blood pressure or pre-eclampsia.

✕ Are expecting twins, triplets or another multiple pregnancy.

✕ Your baby is small for your dates.

✕ Are diagnosed with placenta praevia (one that is low-lying and that covers the cervix) or an incompetent cervix (one prone to early dilatation).

A good workout

The ideal components are a warm-up, which prepares your body to be exercised; aerobic activity to work your heart and lungs; conditioning exercises that strengthen muscle, and cool-down stretches and breathing exercises to return your body to normal.

Pregnant women should try to exercise moderately for at least 30 minutes on most, if not all, days, and to build up their programmes gradually. Try to do a work-out three times a week then progressively increase your number of work-outs. If you find that you get too tired at this level, cut back to three times a week.

Monitor your intensity carefully so that you don't overexert yourself. Because your heart is already pumping about 15 to 20 beats per minute faster than normal, it's essential that you don't push yourself too hard. Learn how to take your pulse and make sure that you exercise within your target heart-rate zone.

Start exercising in short sessions; too much too soon will only lead to sore muscles and exhaustion. For the first few weeks, do 15-minute sessions of aerobic activity at your target heart-rate zone. Increase them only when you're happy at this level.

Warming up and cooling down

These two stages prevent muscle soreness and stiffness. Always include short sessions – 5 to 15 minutes – of warm-up and cool-down activities with any exercise routine. The best warm-up consists of low-intensity, rhythmic activity, such as walking on the spot or stationary cycling, followed by slow, controlled stretches. To cool down effectively, stretch each muscle group in turn. Gentle toning exercises and relaxation or deep-breathing also can be included.

Aerobic activity

Also known as cardiovascular exercise, aerobics involve moving large muscle groups – basically your arms and your legs – for a sustained period of around 15 to 30 minutes. To work effectively during this time, your muscles require a higher oxygen supply than when at rest, and to meet these extra demands, your heart rate and breathing rate have to increase. With repeated exercise, your heart and lungs begin to function more efficiently. Good choices include brisk walking, swimming, or antenatal fitness classes.

Bend and reach aerobic exercise

1 Stand with your feet wider than hip-width and turn out your toes. Lift both arms out to the sides at shoulder height. As you bend both knees, bring your arms into your chest and keep your weight slightly forwards.

2 Straighten your knees, transfer your weight on to your right leg and touch your left foot out to the side, with your leg straight. At the same time, straighten your left arm out to the front and your right arm out to the side at shoulder height.

3 Transfer your weight back to the centre, bend your knees and bring your arms back into your chest. Keep your neck long, shoulders down and chest lifted.

4 Transfer your weight on to your left leg, touch your right foot out, keeping you leg straight, and reverse the arm positions. Repeat.

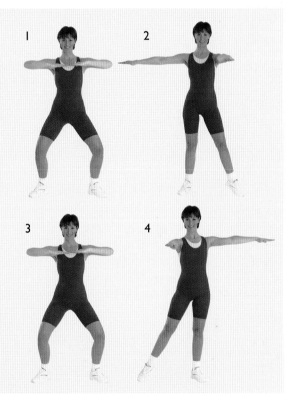

Conditioning exercises

Pregnancy is almost a weightlifting exercise in itself, and because you're carrying those extra pounds, it's more important than ever to keep your muscles strong and toned. To promote muscular strength and endurance (your muscles' ability to perform an exercise repeatedly), you need to isolate groups of muscles and work them against a form of resistance, such as lifting weights at the gym or pushing against water in a water aerobics class.

Before you begin this type of work-out, make sure you know how to perform exercises in a class or use free weights and weight machines correctly; never lift heavy weights during pregnancy – the general rule to follow is to use a weight that you can comfortably lift 12 to 15 times; aim to do two to three sets (12 to 15 repetitions comprise a set) on each muscle but don't get too tired, and keep breathing. When using weights or resistance tools, it's important not to hold your breath. Learn to use your breathing to help you to carry out the exercise: exhale when you exert and inhale when you relax your muscles.

Stop exercising if you experience

✕ Bleeding or any gush of fluid from the vagina.
✕ Unexplained pain in the abdomen.
✕ Persistent headache or changes in vision.
✕ Unexplained faintness or dizziness.
✕ Marked fatigue, heart palpitations, chest pain or excessive breathlessness.

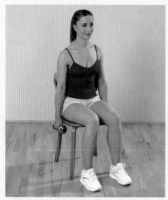
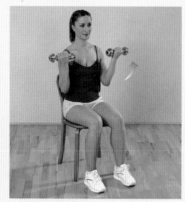
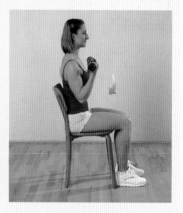

Bicep curl

1 Start in a sitting position. Hold the dumbbells by your sides, palms facing inward. Keep your shoulders, arms, and hands in a straight line, but don't lock your elbows. Keep your abdominals tight to support your back.

2 Exhale as you raise the dumbbells up to your shoulders. Keep your elbows in close to your sides and rotate your forearms as you bring the weights up, until your forearms are vertical and your palms are facing your shoulders. Keep your abdominals tight.

3 Inhale as you steadily lower the weights back to the base position. Keep your arms slightly bent while in the base position.

Finding time to exercise

It is possible to fit exercise into a busy lifestyle.
Checking your posture (see page 193) and performing
pelvic floor exercises (see page 158) can be done
anywhere and as often as possible during the day.
Other things you can do on a regular basis include:

- Taking the stairs rather than a lift, making sure you
  have a breather midway.
- Going for a walk during your lunch break. Try and
  leave heavy bags behind and swing your arms
  gently as you pace briskly.
- Going for a swim on the weekends or perhaps
  joining an evening aqua-natal class. Water can be
  used to give a very effective full body workout.
- Tightening your abdominals before getting into the
  bath or when lying in bed.
- You also can exercise while sitting down at your
  desk, on a bus or train, or at home.

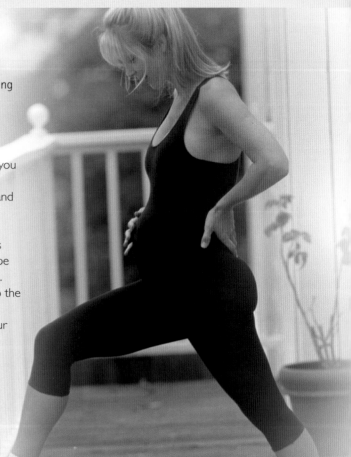

Exercises to do anywhere

The following exercises can be done at home or in the office as long as you are sitting down in a sturdy upright chair.

Neck and shoulders Circle your shoulders slowly back and around, then tip your head gently over to each side. Pause briefly each side.

Chest and spine Slowly squeeze your shoulder blades together to open your chest, and release. Reach your arm down to one side and bend your upper body slowly over; then repeat on the other side. Reach each arm up to the ceiling and hold for a few seconds; repeat.

Lower back and abdominal muscles Tilt your pelvis, curl your back and press your lower back into the chair. Then, tighten your abdominal muscles and lift your baby up and in towards you.

Feet and ankles With one foot off the floor, slowly and gently circle the ankle until it feels looser; repeat with the other foot. Then, lift and lower your heels several times keeping your toes on the floor.

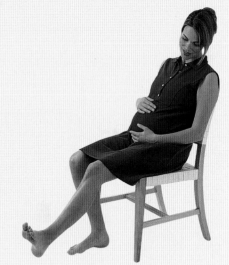

Conserve energy

Use this meditation when you want to

- Relax and take it easy without feeling guilty

- Overcome feelings of tiredness

- Concentrate your energies, particularly if you notice you are easily distracted

How to practise this meditation

Find a comfortable sitting posture that keeps your back straight, rest your hands in your lap, close your eyes, and take a few moments to relax your breathing.

Begin at the top of your head and work down. Note the tension in each area then consciously clench and relaxi it. Ask yourself, 'What is causing my shoulders to feel tired and how can I try to change this?' As you complete the 'scan', consider your priorities. Ask yourself what you need to achieve and on what you need to concentrate your energies now . Although this may take practice, trust your judgment; ask the questions and the answers will come naturally to you.

To improve your energy levels, create a picture of yourself doing the things you want to do and having the energy to do them in a positive, relaxed way. Be flexible and realistic – one day you may just want to survive eight hours at work, while another you may have specific tasks you'd like to fulfil. You can devise a visualisation of your own, or try one of the following:

Imagine energy coursing through your body like a waterfall, from the top of your head, down to your toes. You feel the energy within motivating you to do everything you want, to overcome every obstacle and feel satisfied with each job done.

See yourself in your work environment. You are busy, but can work out what needs to be addressed first and what can wait till later. You are confident and feel happy and rewarded by your work.

mini meditation
Slowing down

Choose an everyday chore like getting dressed and perform every associated activity consciously slower, leaving yourself extra time so you don't feel hurried. Focus closely on every movement you make. Notice the pace at which you open the wardrobe and pull out a hanger. Enjoy the passing sensations – the feel of the fabric, the sound of a zipper being fastened, the smell of a freshly laundered shirt. Concentrate on the present, not others things you 'should' be doing.

Antenatal checks

Throughout your pregnancy, you and your baby will be closely monitored to make sure that everything is progressing as it should. Your healthcare provider will also want to ensure that you are prepared for childbirth and parenthood.

Your first visit

For many women, this is around weeks 6 to 8 and will probably be to confirm the news that you're pregnant.

The 'booking' appointment

This should take place between weeks 8 and 10 and will include a full physical examination. You will also have blood drawn to test for your blood type and rhesus status, to ascertain your blood cell count, and to check whether you are immune to Rubella (German measles) and syphilis. Other blood tests can check immunity to hepatitis B and whether you carry the HIV virus. Your urine will be checked for signs of diabetes and your blood pressure for signs of elevation. Your medical history will be taken and your height and weight measured. An ultrasound may be given to confirm your due date. You will be given your maternity record, which details the results of all tests carried out during your pregnancy.

Schedule of visits

After that, your schedule of visits will vary depending on your healthcare provider and medical needs. With a normal, low-risk pregnancy, you'll probably have monthly visits until weeks 28 to 32, when you'll start to go for more frequent visits, every one or two weeks. At each visit, it's likely that your blood pressure will be taken, your urine will be tested for protein and perhaps glucose and the baby's size and position will be checked. The baby's heart rate may be monitored from week 16 onwards. You should use your visits to discuss with your healthcare provider how you're coping and whether you have any pregnancy-related complaints or concerns.

Date/Time	Place	Procedure

EARLY TESTS

These fall into two categories. The first are screening tests, which are non-invasive and pose no threat to the baby. They include ultrasound and blood tests. The other, or diagnostic tests, involve removing either tissue or fluid from the amniotic sac to determine whether there are chromosomal abnormalities, as is the case with Down's syndrome. Chorionic villus sampling and amniocentesis are the two main tests, but only the former is performed in the first trimester.

Ultrasound

In a painfree procedure that causes no harm to a woman or her baby in the short or long term, sound waves and their echoes create a picture of the uterus and a developing baby. Ultrasound scans are performed either transvaginally, using a probe that inserts into the vagina, or trans-abdominally, using a transducer that is moved across the mother's abdomen. Doppler ultrasound scanning traces the blood flow between the placenta and your baby through the umbilical cord.

Scans performed before 8 to 10 weeks of pregnancy are usually done vaginally because this gives a clearer picture, being much closer to the baby at this stage of pregnancy. Although it's understandable to worry, there is no evidence that the probe can harm you or your baby.

Scans later in pregnancy are usually done transabdominally since the baby is clearly visible in the abdomen by then. Gel is spread over the abdominal skin and the transducer is moved on the gel. The sound waves travel through liquid such as the amniotic fluid but are reflected (bounced back) by more solid structures such as the heart, brain and uterine wall. The quality of the pictures depends on several variables including the quality of the scanning machine; the training and skills of the technician; the length of time for which you are scanned; the way your baby is lying, and whether you are very overweight, or there is a lot of scar tissue.

Early/dating scan

This is usually carried out between 11-14 weeks of pregnancy. A nuchal transparency scan will form part of the examination.

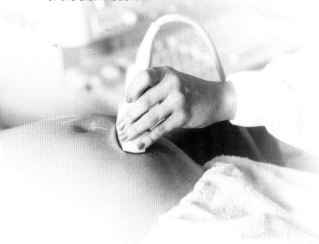

This ultrasound will

- Locate the pregnancy – is it in the uterus?
- Establish an accurate date of delivery. Scans done before 20 weeks give a much clearer indication of the delivery date than later scans.
- Check the number of babies. If you have twins (or more), the appearance of the membrane separating the babies and the position of the placenta can show whether the babies share one placenta or have one each.
- Check the uterus and ovaries. The size and shape of the uterus and appearance of the cervix will be assessed, and if you have fibroids (common benign overgrowths of the muscle wall of the uterus), they can be measured.
- Assess the risk of Down's syndrome. The nuchal translucency screening test involves measuring a special fluid-filled area behind the baby's neck. If this is thicker than average, the risk of Down's syndrome is increased, and you will be offered further testing, including blood tests, amniocentesis and CVS. Bear in mind that even if your risk is higher, there is still a good chance that the baby is absolutely normal.

Blood tests

Your blood will be tested to screen for anaemia, to check your blood group and rhesus factor status, and to assess your immunity or previous exposure to certain infections. Currently all women are tested for rubella, Hepatitis B, syphilis and HIV. You will have pre-test counselling for all these checks.

Diagnostic blood tests also may be offered if you or your partner have a history of an inherited disease, or if there is a better-than-average chance that you and your partner could be carrying a defective gene for a particular disorder, even though there is no known history of the condition in your immediate family. Blood tests also are used to identify diseases that can be passed on from only one carrier parent, such as haemophilia, or from an affected parent, as in the case of Huntington's.

There are specific substances in the maternal blood, which have come from the baby and the placenta, that are raised with Down's syndrome and also with some neural tube defects. These are alpha-fetoprotein (AFP), human chorionic gonadotropin (HCG), a placental substance (PAPP-A), uE3 and inhibin A. Soon, all women who want to be screened will be offered the combined test (NT, hCG and PAPP-A) and the integrated test (NT, hCG and PAPP-A, AFP, uE3, inhibin A) and the serum integrated test (Papp-A and hCG, AFP, ue3, inhibin A) from 11 to 14 weeks.

These tests only give an idea of risk, but will pick up more than 75 per cent of women whose babies are at risk (greater than 1 in 250). An actual diagnosis can be achieved only by looking at the baby's chromosomes. This is done by two methods –chorionic villus sampling (CVS) and amniocentesis (see page 148).

Determing Rh status is important. If you are rhesus negative and your baby rhesus positive, you can develop antibodies, which can be dangerous to your next rhesus positive baby.

Chorionic villus sampling (CVS)

CVS may be offered if a fetal abnormality is suspected. Typically done between 10 and 13 weeks of pregnancy, it means that if an abnormality is present, and pregnancy termination is an option, termination can be done earlier, which can be physically and emotionally easier for the mother.

Chorionic villi are placental tissue that contain the same chromosomes and genetic make-up as your developing baby. Some is withdrawn through a hollow needle inserted through the abdomen – transabdominal CVS, or through a flexible catheter inserted through the cervix – transcervical CVS. Ultrasound is used to guide the doctor to the right location and to avoid injury to the baby as the procedure is performed. The location of the placenta within the uterus and the general shape and position of the uterus itself determines whether CVS is performed through the abdomen or the cervix. The tissue is then processed in a laboratory and a karyotype (a picture of the chromosomes) is prepared. The results are available in about seven days, although it can take two to three weeks for a full report.

Regardless of whether the CVS is performed through the cervix or the abdomen, neither method is riskier than the other, although having an invasive test always slightly raises the risk of miscarriage. Studies show that the experience of the person performing the procedure is important in reducing this risk.

Some vaginal bleeding may occur after CVS and should not be a cause for concern, although you should report it to your healthcare provider if it lasts for three or more days. There is also a very slight risk of infection, so you should tell your healthcare provider if you have a fever in the days following the procedure.

Chorionic villi are tiny, fingerlike pieces of tissue that make up the placenta. They develop from cells arising out of the fertilized egg.

Find peace of mind

Use this meditation when you want to

- Feel in control of your emotions

- Accept changes that will inevitably happen

- Cope with sudden tearful outbursts

- Deal with worries or feelings of uncertainty

How to practise this meditation

Music is wonderful for calming turbulent emotions and soothing fears. Meditation heightens all your senses so an aural focus is a particularly good way to still confused or conflicting thoughts, and help you put things into perspective.

If you feel yourself mentally chasing your own tail, take time out and find a place where you can be alone and listen to a favourite piece of music. This way you can create an oasis of tranquillity anywhere – even if this just means sitting in the car with your eyes shut, the doors closed, and the music playing. You can use any type of non-vocal music: choose something that is meaningful to you – uplifting, inspirational or calming, depending on your mood.

As you listen, focus on how the music resonates in your body and what effect it has on your physical state. Concentrate on the fact that being calm is doing your body good too. If the music arouses mental associations and images, accept them and use them to extend your meditation. However, don't allow yourself to be distracted: ask yourself every so often if you are still following the music and gently bring yourself back if your mind wanders. You may also wish to use an affirmation to support the positive feelings that the music arouses. Try one of the following affirmations, or adapt one to suit your mood:

- I accept myself as I am
- I am aware of what comes into my mind and keeps me from feeling peaceful
- My family will be happy and healthy

If you find that you are distracted by negative thoughts, try thinking of them as 'roadblocks' to peace of mind. Use the affirmation to acknowledge these mental obstacles and think positively about yourself to move beyond them. Spend a few quiet moments at the end of the meditation to appreciate how your anxiety has been quieted.

Twins

Discovering that you're going to have more than one baby can come as a shock. Some women, especially if they're a twin themselves or if they've already had one baby, have an inkling that 'something's up' but can't quite believe it until they see conclusive proof on the ultrasound scan. Multiple pregnancies are diagnosed by an early ultrasound scan; one at 12 to 14 weeks will identify how many babies are present, and may reveal whether the twins are identical.

This early 'warning' enables you and your antenatal team to plan a specially tailored schedule of tests and check-ups and allows time for you and your partner to adjust emotionally, so that you can get on with the practicalities that preparation for two babies requires. Being prepared helps to reduce extra anxiety about the approaching births, because you feel more in control and ready to respond as necessary.

You may want to contact the Twins and Multiple Births Association (TAMBA) for specific advice and information. You'll discover all sorts of handy hints and tips from chatting to other parents of twins and listening to their stories.

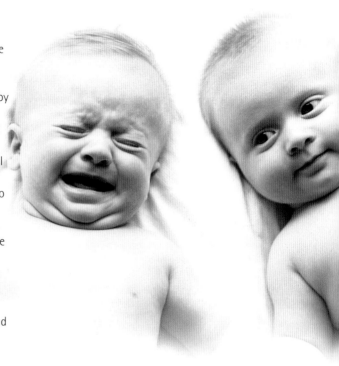

What to expect

Carrying twins (or more) can be much more complicated than carrying a singleton, so your medical team will want to keep a close eye on how everything is progressing. You may experience exaggerated pregnancy symptoms – compared with carrying a singleton – so severe morning sickness and extreme tiredness in the early days could be clues that something is different. Your antenatal care will involve:

More frequent check-ups

At which your blood pressure and urine protein will be checked more regularly for signs of pre-eclampsia (see page 239) and anaemia (see page 235).

More ultrasound scans

Because it's difficult to monitor the growth and development of twins with a simple examination, your healthcare provider will want accurate and regular updates on how your babies are getting on in their uterine world. If your twins are nonidentical you'll probably have a scan every four weeks, or every two weeks if they're identical twins, as complications are more common.

Premature labour and early delivery

Babies are born early – by week 37 – in 50 per cent of twin pregnancies. Contact your healthcare provider immediately if you have any signs of pain, bleeding or watery vaginal discharge.

A hospital delivery

Although you can have twins normally, if the first baby is head first, keep in mind that it's not unusual for women carrying twins to require delivery by Caesarean (see page 292).

Extra maternity leave

If you work, both your tiredness and your increased need for rest may mean you have to stop working earlier on in your pregnancy and take more time off.

COMBATTING EARLY SIDE EFFECTS

Most women suffer from tiredness and many from morning sickness, heartburn or tender breasts during the first trimester, but it is important not to let these physical discomforts dominate the early months. Try to think positively: these ailments are your body's natural response to the changes happening within it and signs that your pregnancy is progressing well. You also can think of them as proof that there is a new life growing within you. You may find this difficult, especially if you have very much wanted to be pregnant and now find you feel sick all the time, but be reassured that these complaints won't last forever: by the second trimester you will be glowing with health and energy.

A strong belief that you will be well can have an enormous effect on how you feel; it can help you remain relaxed during discomfort, and foster a positive attitude toward your symptoms. Meditating can physically relieve many complaints by regulating your breathing and other body functions and there are other natural remedies and solutions that can help you overcome their effects.

Morning sickness

About half of all pregnant women experience morning sickness to some degree; most find their symptoms are worst during the first trimester and improve considerably, if not completely, thereafter.

The exact cause of morning sickness remains something of a mystery, but experts believe it is linked to the high levels of hormones travelling through the maternal bloodstream, and particularly of progesterone, which is produced within the ovaries during the first 12–14 weeks of pregnancy. Blood sugar levels are also affected during pregnancy and if they fall, for instance after a long evening without food or if you're not eating enough, this can cause nausea, which may or may not be accompanied by vomiting.

Although it often occurs in the morning, the nausea can last all day. If your queasiness gets out of control – you lose weight, can't keep down food or liquids, become dizzy or faint, consult your caregiver. In the most severe (but rare) cases, severe vomiting can lead to hospitalisation due to loss of fluids.

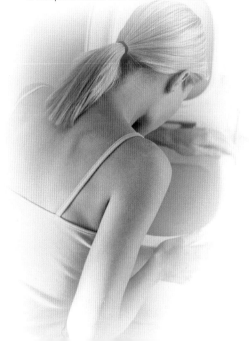

What you can do to help

- Eat little and often.
- Avoid spicy, strong-smelling foods.
- Eat high-carbohydrate foods such as dry toast, potatoes and cereals.
- Try a ginger-based drink – ginger ale or tea – or snack on ginger biscuits.
- Avoid cigarette smoke and rich perfumes.
- Keep plain crackers by the bedside and eat some before you get out of bed.
- Try acupressure wrist bands.
- Try pressing the accupressure point P6 (in the middle of the inside of the forearm, two or three fingerwidths up from the wrist crease. Use vibrating pressure for 20 seconds.

Dizziness and fainting

Feeling light-headed is common and in the early stages, it may occur as your blood flow strives to catch up with your increased circulation. Later on, dizziness can be a result of the uterus pressing on large blood vessels. Low blood-sugar levels, low blood pressure, getting up too quickly or becoming overheated can all contribute to dizzy spells.

Fainting during pregnancy is rare, but if you do faint it's because the flow of blood to your brain is reduced temporarily. This will not harm your baby. Report fainting to your healthcare provider right away as this may be a sign of severe anaemia.

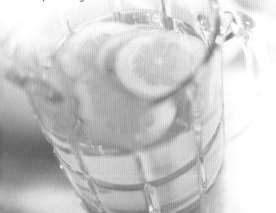

What you can do to help

- Get up slowly from sitting or lying down so that the blood has time to flow to your brain.
- When you're lying down, rest on one side or the other whenever possible; don't lie flat on your back.
- Drink plenty of liquids – dizziness can be a sign of dehydration – and don't avoid salt.
- Eat complex carbohydrates at every meal or try eating smaller, more frequent meals to maintain your blood-sugar levels.
- Carry raisins, a piece of fruit or some cream crackers in your bag for a quick blood-sugar lift.
- If you feel too warm, get some fresh air and loosen your clothes around the neck and waist.
- If you feel faint, try to increase the circulation to your brain by sitting with your head between your knees or lying down with your feet higher than your head.

Tiredness

In the first three months of pregnancy, your body has a hard time keeping up physically with the mental excitement you're experiencing. Once the first flush of elation is over, you may feel totally exhausted and just want to curl up and sleep for hours. This is to be expected: your body is having to cope with enormous changes, even if you are not yet aware of them, which means it's working a lot harder than usual. Fatigue may be a side effect of the dramatic rise in hormone levels. You'll probably find that your exhaustion goes away around weeks 12 to 14. As fatigue lessens, you'll begin to feel more energetic and almost normal, until about 30 to 34 weeks when you may feel tired again. At this point, part of the fatigue is due to carrying around extra weight. Women often find their second or third pregnancies more tiring than their first, because they have to care for other children.

What you can do to help

- Try to be realistic about what you can do, and don't feel guilty about what you can't get done. Prioritise your tasks, doing only what is essential. Let some of your commitments drop.
- Get as much rest as you can by sitting with your feet up during the evenings and going to bed earlier.
- Whenever possible, let other people help with household chores and other responsibilities. This is especially important if you already have children and can't just put your feet up when you feel like it.
- Make sure you are eating a healthy pregnancy diet and avoid caffeine and sweets, which will give you a quick energy lift and then leave your body feeling more fatigued as the blood-sugar level drops.
- Do some gentle exercise every day.
- Practise the conserve energy meditation on page 116.

Overcome early physical complaints

Use this meditation when you want to	How to practise this meditation
• Dispel fears that you'll never stop feeling sick • Remain relaxed, in spite of physical discomfort • Accept your complaints, not fight them • Free your mind to focus on more positive aspects of your pregnancy	Choose a comfortable place with plenty of cushions. If you are feeling sick, uncomfortable or your breasts are very tender, wear loose clothing and lie down to do this exercise. Focusing on your breathing can be particularly useful in overcoming nausea. Begin by breathing normally and count each out-breath until you reach ten. Then repeat the process, counting the in-breaths. This will help you concentrate your mind on your breathing and away from your symptoms. As you focus on each breath, think of a time when you felt wonderful and energetic. Concentrate on feeling good and let the feeling wash over you, dispersing any discomfort.

Use a visualisation to turn your discomfort into a positive experience or to rid yourself of it completely. When you are in doubt or pain, it may help to recall the story about Buddha who, while sitting in meditation during an attack from an enemy army, turned the missiles falling all around him into harmless, sweet-scented flowers. Personalise one of the following to suit your needs:

If you're suffering from morning sickness, visualise a television screen showing your body. Notice that the pain-free areas are shining with a white light. Then concentrate on those aching parts you want to heal. Imagine the light slowly expanding so that gradually your whole body is bathed in it and you can rejoice in your healthy, glowing body.

If you're suffering from tender breasts, imagine that your baby is born. You are holding your baby to your breast and the tenderness you are feeling is because your baby is feeding and you are the sole provider of his or her daily needs. Your baby only has eyes for you and is warm and secure in your arms.

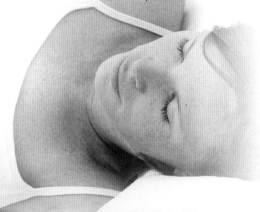

Fears and anxieties

The pleasure of pregnancy can sometimes be marred by fears and worries such as that of losing a child. Antenatal testing, too, is a common source of worry even though it is designed to detect problems early so that a baby has the best chance of being born healthy.

Some mothers have concerns about the impact of their lifestyles on their babies, particularly if they smoked, drank alcohol or were exposed to environmental hazards before they realized they were pregnant. In these cases, the best way to limit anxiety is to adjust your lifestyle so that you provide a healthy environment for your baby.

Some women who are conscious of their figures feel disturbed by their increasing size during pregnancy. If you begin to feel like this, try not to be embarrassed about your bump: you aren't getting fat, you're growing a baby. As the months go by, you'll come to terms with your changing shape. At first, you may feel frustrated that there's nothing to see. In the second or third month, as your clothes begin to feel tight, you may experience impatience, because you're no longer the shape you were, but neither are you recognizably pregnant. Around the fourth month, you'll probably be relieved that your protruding tummy is clearly visible. Discussing concerns with your healthcare provider should also put your mind at ease.

Miscarriage

This is a worry common to many mothers-to-be and is connected with anxiety about having a healthy baby.

These fears may be especially acute if you have experienced a miscarriage in the past; in this case it is even more important to relax and stay calm during the early months of pregnancy if you are to enjoy it fully.

A confident attitude can help you tackle your fears and remain relaxed during the first three months of pregnancy when you are at the highest risk of miscarriage. If you have lost a previous pregnancy, it may be difficult to keep calm, but remember that the majority of women who have had a miscarriage go on to have normal, healthy pregnancies.

Miscarriage occurs when the fetus spontaneously aborts before the twenty-eighth week. Usually due to an abnormality, it is most common in the first few weeks of pregnancy, and frequently happens before the pregnancy has been confirmed or even suspected. It may help to think of miscarriage as nature's way of ending a pregnancy that, for whatever reason, cannot go full term. It is important, therefore, not to blame yourself – doctors say that if a miscarriage is going to happen there is almost nothing you can do about it.

Danger signs

If you experience vaginal bleeding at any stage during your pregnancy, especially if it is accompanied by pain, you should

✓ Seek prompt medical attention.

✓ Go to bed or lie down somewhere comfortable and wait for the doctor.

✓ Prop your feet up on some pillows to keep your legs and hips raised.

✓ Use a cold compress or fan to keep cool. Above all, remember that although vaginal bleeding occurs in a quarter of all pregnancies, most proceed healthily to full term.

✗ Not take any alcohol, painkillers or any other medication until you have consulted a doctor.

Cope with the fear of miscarriage

Use this meditation when you want to

- Calm any worries about losing your baby

- Acknowledge and express your feelings about a previous miscarriage

- Learn to look to the future rather than the past

How to practise this meditation

Choose a place you find reassuring, where you feel tranquil and secure, and find a comfortable position that allows you to breathe freely and easily. Spend a few moments thinking about your body and consciously make tiny adjustments to your posture to ease any areas of tension.

Allow the muscles in your chest and abdomen to loosen to give your breath room to move around your body. Let your breathing be spontaneous – think about it without trying to breathe 'correctly'. The way in which you breathe reflects your emotional state. When you are feeling over-emotional, your stress levels rise and your breathing becomes shallow and hurried, which in turn increases your sense of strain.

Conversely, as your breathing slows and becomes more relaxed, your mind will become calm and the tension will ease out of your body.

Keep focused by counting each inhalation. If your concentration wanders and you lose count, gently bring your attention back to your breathing without getting annoyed. If you feel sleepy, concentrate more intently on the sensations in your body – how has your breathing changed? What emotions are you experiencing?

As you relax the physical and mental defences of everyday life, your fears and grief may surface. Acknowledge painful or fearful emotions but let them leave your body with each exhalation. Use this time of quietness to say good-bye if you have experienced a previous loss. Now focus on the future and concentrate your thoughts on the new baby within. Put your hands on your belly and visualise the comforting protective environment of your uterus. Imagine all the nutrients your growing fetus needs travelling across the placenta and down the umbilical cord from you to your baby. Feel how attached the two of you are, and reassure yourself that everything is fine.

Impending parenthood

You may feel distinctly nervous about this untried role. If marriage or moving in with your partner seemed a huge step, the addition of a baby can be an even more momentous change. You may fear a loss of independence or experience sudden panics that your partner may not want to be as involved as you would like. Your partner may be concerned about being left out after the new arrival or how you will manage financially on one salary.

It takes time for an individual to grow into a parent. Being a good mother or father certainly doesn't happen as soon as your baby is born. Pregnancy, besides being a period of waiting, is a time of preparation for parenthood. Talk to other parents, and use every opportunity to get close to newborns. The best way to learn is by hands-on experience, so ask to baby-sit for a friend with a baby. Practise holding, changing and playing with him or her. Your friend may be kind enough to return the favour after your baby is born and you need a break.

Make sure, too, you involve your partner as much as you can. Try and see yourselves as a team, building a secure environment for your child.

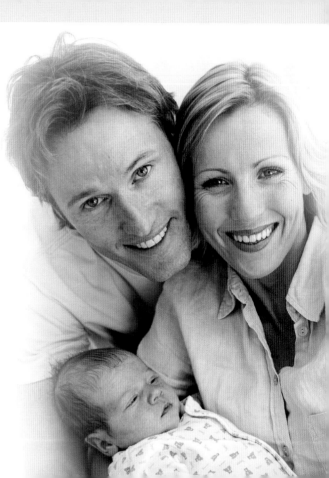

Single motherhood

For many women, the early signs of pregnancy are a very exciting time – but this period can also be scary and isolating. As a single mother-to-be, you may be worried about your ability to cope. You will really be looking within yourself, pulling on resources and emotions that you may not have known you had, and learning to be strong for the sake of your child and whatever the future brings. Bear in mind, however, that being a single mother does not mean you are alone. Lean on your family and friends for the support you need. If you don't have a family to fall back on, local or internet-based self-help organisations can put you in touch with other single parents and provide emotional and practical support. You also may like to think about choosing a particular person who can accompany you on your antenatal check-ups and later act as your birth partner. A trained or experienced birth helper is an option. You can hire a doula or a monitrice, whose services usually include visits before and after delivery, as well as at-home support. Ask your healthcare provider for more information and recommendations.

It is important that you use your energy positively, concentrate on the happy aspects of life, and allow yourself to let go of the things that are really not important. Meditation will strengthen your belief in yourself and help quell your doubts.

Bringing a child into the world on your own is something very special; it takes great courage and strength. Celebrate this courage and think positively about your pregnancy. You will have a very intimate relationship with your child, who will be dependent on you for love, guidance and protection throughout his or her life.

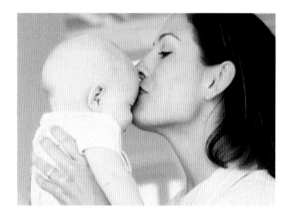

Face the prospect of single motherhood

Use this meditation when you want to

- Quell feelings of loneliness

- Find courage to feel positive about the future

- Boost your self-confidence and believe in the strength of your convictions

- Find inner peace and contentment

How to practise this meditation

Choose a place where you feel secure and comfortable and that inspires you with feelings of capability and courage. Take a few moments to become calm, using a technique that works for you – such as counting your breaths – before focusing on a visualisation. Close your eyes and concentrate on all the things you can do as a mother, now and in the years to come. If you are experiencing hurt, resentment or anger, let these feelings enter your mind but then let them pass.

Visualisations can help you to love yourself and accept the situation you are in now. If you are wondering whether you have done the right thing, use a visualisation to accept that this is the road you are on and that it is the route to a positive life ahead.

Imagine yourself walking along a beautiful, tree-lined road. You are walking slowly but assuredly. Occasionally there is a pothole or a rock to climb over or around, but you see these obstacles coming and easily deal with them. You are not tired walking, but full of energy, with a spring in your step, because you know you are walking towards something beautiful and eternally fulfilling.

mini meditation
At times of self-doubt

Chanting a mantra under your breath when you are alone, or silently if you're in company is useful when you are struck by fears. Choose a short, meaningful phrase that has affirmative associations for you and is easy to remember (see also page 20). Bring it to mind whenever you feel the need to reassure yourself. If you are religious, try a phrase with spiritual significance, or use:

- Healthy am I. Happy am I. Holy am I.
- We two are special.

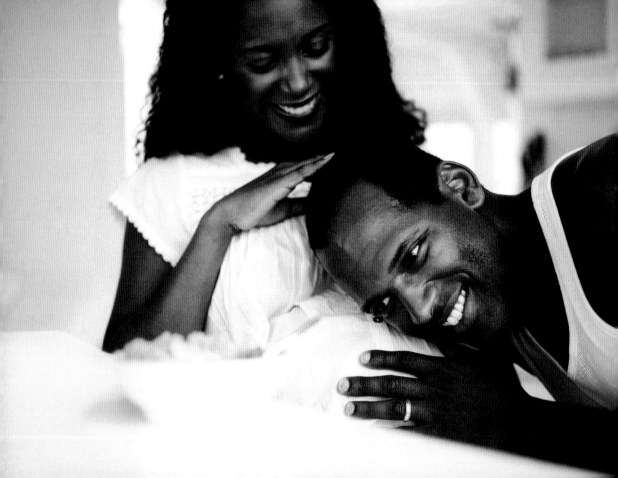

Chapter 3

The second trimester

WELL AND TRULY PREGNANT

This trimester represents the next sixteen weeks of your pregnancy. It is often the easiest and most enjoyable of the three trimesters. You'll find you're less tired and have more energy to deal with all the changes taking place – so make the most of this wonderful time! At the beginning you will notice that your abdomen is becoming more rounded and your waistline is starting to disappear. But by week twenty-eight, your waistline will have completely gone, you'll have probably gained around 6 kg and have a beautiful big bump in front of you. Nurture your baby and yourself by eating well, getting plenty of rest and looking after your body to prevent problems such as backache and swollen ankles.

Antenatal checks

You and your baby will continue to be monitored regularly, with appointments scheduled at around 4-weekly intervals. These visits are less detailed and lengthy than your first, and will involve fewer checks. Routine tests include taking your blood pressure to check for signs of pre-eclampsia or hypertension (also characterised by swollen feet and hands and the presence of protein in the urine); urine samples to check for signs of urinary infection or the onset of diabetes (which can temporarily occur during pregnancy) and blood tests to check for anaemia. You also will be offered an opportunity to discuss any pregnancy-related complaints or concerns that you may have.

Don't be tempted to skip appointments because you feel all right - regular checks are needed because they are the best way to keep an eye on you and your developing baby. If, for any reason, you can't make an appointment, make sure you reschedule.

At about 16 weeks of pregnancy, you will have another visit during which your blood test results from your booking appointment will be discussed and you

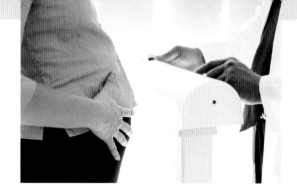

may be able to hear your baby's heartbeat using a Sonicaid (a handheld ultrasound monitor). You may be offered a blood test for Down's syndrome at this time.

At about 20 weeks your appointment may include an ultrasound scan to check the baby's anatomy and growth (see page 146).

At each visit, your healthcare provider will palpate your abdomen and measure your fundal height. This measurement is the distance from the top of your uterus to your pelvic bone. It lengthens as your baby grows and so gives an estimate of his size for age. If your healthcare provider thinks your baby is either too big or too small, you'll probably be referred for an ultrasound scan for a more accurate measurement.

Date/Time	Place	Procedure

Diagnostic tests

You are probably feeling more at ease now that your pregnancy is well established and the uncertainty of the first twelve weeks is over. It is around this time that you may have certain antenatal tests to ensure that you are in good health and that all is progressing well with your baby. Several different tests are available; these can give an indication of problems, such as spina bifida, but not all are definitive. If you are uncertain about the risks involved, discuss the necessity of each test with your doctor.

Most pregnancies are perfectly normal, but having tests can be stressful, particularly if you feel you may have cause for concern, perhaps because of your age or family medical history. In turn, this stress can affect your wellbeing and although your baby won't be unduly affected by short-term stress, he or she will be aware of the tension in your body. If you find yourself lying awake at night, worrying about undergoing your antenatal tests, try to look at them as positive procedures, which are aimed at helping you and your baby to have a healthy and successful pregnancy. The meditation on page 150 also can help to reduce stress.

Anomaly ultrasound scan

This is performed at around 16 to 22 weeks. It is much more detailed than the dating scan and checks :

Fetal anatomy All the baby's organs including the brain and spinal cord, heart, chest cavity, stomach, face, kidneys and bladder, and arms and legs are checked. Even the number of toes and fingers can be counted, if the scan suggests an abnormality, you may be referred for an MRI (magnetic resonance imaging) scan.

Gestational age The maturity of the fetus.

Amount of amniotic fluid To check it is adequate.

Growth rate The length of the baby is measured from the head to the bottom – the crown-rump length.

Location of the placenta The position, size and function of the placenta is checked. If the placenta is low-lying, near or across the cervix, you will be rescanned later in pregnancy. If, later on, the placenta or its blood vessels are seen to cover the cervix, you will need to have a Caesarean. The placenta can be investigated further using colour doppler scanning to trace the blood flow through the umbilical cord.

Baby's gender After 16 weeks it is often easy to see if you have a boy or a girl. Don't depend completely on this though!

Blood tests

There are specific substances in the maternal blood, which have come from the baby and the placenta, which are raised with Down's syndrome and also with some neural tube defects. Soon the following tests will be available to all women who want to be screened:

From 14 to 20 weeks The quadruple test (hCG, AFP, uE3, inhibin A).

From 14 to 20 weeks The integrated test (NT, hCG and PAPP-A, AFP, uE3, inhibin A) and the serum integrated test (Papp-A and hCG, AFP, ue£, inhibin A).

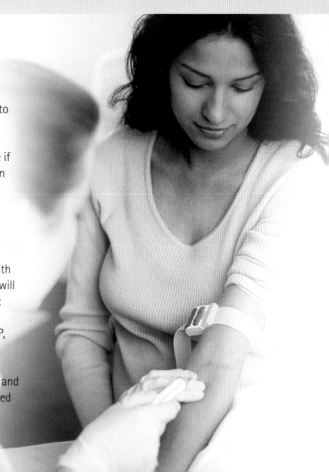

Amniocentesis

This test for genetic abnormalities is usually done at 15 to 20 weeks. It primarily tests to see that 23 pairs of chromosome are present and that their structures are normal. It doesn't routinely test for all possible genetic diseases or structural abnormalities.

Amniocentesis also may be used to test for specific genetic disorders for which the baby is known to be a high risk – for example, cystic fibrosis, Tay-Sachs disease, or Huntington's disease.

Amniocentesis will be offered if you had a high-risk result from other tests for Down's syndrome.

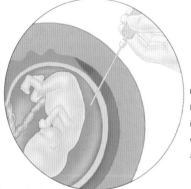

Cells that contain a baby's **DNA** are shed into the amniotic fluid, which can be collected and analyzed.

How it's performed

The procedure is usually carried out by a specialist obstetrician who will use ultrasound to identify a 'pocket' of amniotic fluid away from the baby. A thin needle will be inserted through the abdomen and uterine wall into the amniotic sac. About 15 to 20 cc (one to two tablespoons) of amniotic fluid will be withdrawn, after which the needle is removed. An amniocentesis needle is very thin, so any discomfort should be minimal.

The procedure only lasts about one to two minutes, although it may feel longer. It's mildly uncomfortable but not terribly painful. Most women report that it isn't as bad as they expected it to be. Generally a slight, brief cramping sensation is felt as the needle goes into the uterus, followed by a strange pulling sensation as the fluid is withdrawn through the needle. While some doctors choose to give local anaesthesia, others feel that the discomfort caused by the injection of the anaesthetic agent isn't worth the benefit. After all, the anaesthesia only numbs the skin, and doesn't numb the uterus where any discomfort will be felt. Afterwards, your doctor may advise that you rest for one to two days and avoid strenuous activity and sex during this period.

Risks and side effects

There is a small risk of miscarriage with this test. After the procedure some women experience cramping for several hours. The best treatment for this is rest. You may experience a little leakage of amniotic fluid through the vagina – no more than a teaspoonful. A small leakage that then stops is usually alright, but if you experience a gush of fluid, call your doctor immediately. You may also experience spotting which lasts a few days.

Many parents worry that having an amniocentesis will harm the baby, but the chance of this happening is extremely rare, given the use of ultrasound guidance.

Results

Results are usually available in 1 to 2 weeks as cells taken during the amniocentesis must be incubated and cultured. If there is a high suspicion of a chromosomal abnormality like Down's syndrome, trisomy 18 or trisomy 13, some laboratories will perform a preliminary, rapid test called a Fluorescent in Situ Hybridization (FISH), which takes 24 to 48 hours for a result. A FISH isn't a final result, and only tests for certain common chromosomal abnormalities.

Down's syndrome

This chromosomal disorder, also known as 21 trisomy, results when an individual has all or part of an extra 21st chromosome. Often it is associated with some impairment of cognitive ability and physical growth as well as a characteristic facial appearance in which the eyes are almond shaped due to an epicanthic fold of the eyelid. People born with Down's syndrome have a higher risk for congenital heart defects, gastroesophageal reflux disease, recurrent ear infections, obstructive sleep apnea, and thyroid dysfunctions. The risk of a baby having Down's syndrome can be estimated by a combination of ultrasound examination (nuchal transparency screening, see page 121) and serum testing. The risk of having a Down's syndrome baby increases with age. 1 in 2000 babies born to 20-year-old mothers will be born with the condition compared with 1 in 100 babies born to 40-year-old mothers.

Relieve anxiety

Use this meditation when you want to

- Face anxieties about your baby's wellbeing

- Master fears about having antenatal tests

- Keep the jitters at bay when you're waiting for test results

How to practise this meditation

It can be useful to combine both a full meditation and a 'mini' one on the days when you have a test. This way you can calm and prepare yourself before you set off, then practise a simple technique on the way to the clinic, in the waiting room, or even during a scan to encourage positive thoughts and give you continuous inner balance and tranquillity.

For both the main and mini meditations, focus first on your breathing. Notice how it begins naturally to slow down and regulate as each breath exhales from your body. Count each out-breath – say up to ten – before starting again, to keep you focused.

For your main meditation, continue this breathing for fifteen minutes, with both hands placed flat on your abdomen so that you feel in touch with your baby. You also may choose a mantra, a particular word that conveys the positive feelings you have about yourself and your baby. You could use a word such as 'Calm' or 'Love', or the traditional Hindu mantra, 'Om'.

mini meditation
Calming down

Start by focusing on your breathing (see opposite) then once it has calmed down, think about your bump. Look at it a couple of times and sense its firm roundness. Let your surroundings fade into the background and feel time slow down. Allow your body to relax and your shoulders to drop. Imagine how your bump would feel now if you were gently stroking it – the sensation of your hand on your smooth, bare skin. Then gently bring yourself back into the present and be aware of how calm you are now feeling.

Healthy eating

At this stage in your pregnancy, nausea often diminishes so you may start to enjoy eating again and feel more energetic. If you have regained your appetite, enjoy eating a varied diet as this is as important as ever for you and your baby.

Although it can be tempting to overeat, unnecessary weight gain can be difficult to shift later. Eating sensibly will curb hunger, provide you and your baby with the nutrients you need, and help you to manage your weight. When you are tempted to munch your way through a packet of biscuits, investigate the fruit bowl instead. An apple or pear will release sugars much more slowly into the bloodstream and will help prevent the peaks and troughs caused by eating for instant energy. If biscuits are really all you want, eat some fruit first and then eat one or two biscuits. That way your craving for biscuits is met (in part), you have eaten some vitamins, you have energy for later, and you will have eaten fewer empty calories.

Make your life easier by keeping a supply of fruit, vegetables, bread, nuts and seeds at home and to snack on at work.

Even if you are eating a varied diet, make sure you don't undo your hard work. For example, drinking tea or coffee at mealtimes can reduce the amount of iron your body can obtain from the food you eat. Leave a gap of at least 30 minutes after eating before drinking tea or coffee.

Eating a large amount of wholegrain foods (brown rice, wholemeal pasta and bread) is good for most people, but, in excess, can reduce the amount of calcium, iron and zinc your body can absorb.

During pregnancy your metabolic rate increases by around 20 per cent. This means that even when you are resting, your body feels much hotter than usual. If you do feel over-heated, you should drink more water than usual to replace the additional fluids that you are losing through perspiration.

Second trimester needs

Although your baby is fully formed, she needs a range of nutrients to support her development. Some of the most important nutrients at this time are essential fatty acids, which are vital for the development of her brain and eyes, iodine and vitamin D. Calcium is important for nerve transmission and muscle contraction, as well as for healthy teeth and bones.

Fatty acids, iodine and vitamin D

Fish and seafood (but make sure you read page 59) are the best dietary sources of the omega 3 fatty acids DHA and EPA. They also are excellent sources of iodine, which the thyroid gland needs to function properly. If you don't eat fish, your doctor may advise you to take a supplement.

Your baby also needs a good supply of vitamin D and calcium to help make healthy teeth and bones. Fish also is the main dietary source of vitamin D but you can get it from egg yolks, milk, butter and fortified breakfast cereals if you cannot eat fish. It also is recommended that you take a 10 mcg supplement of vitamin D each day because although sunshine is synthesised to make the vitamin, levels in the UK are low. If abroad, moderate exposure to the sun also generates vitamin D, although this should be balanced against increasing your risk of skin cancer. Just half-

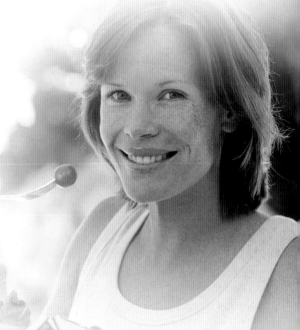

an-hour a day is enough to get the vitamin D you need, so try not to overdo it. Wearing sun protection lotion is essential for the health of your skin, and will not stop your body absorbing vitamin D.

Calcium

As you are supplying calcium to your baby for her skeleton, make sure that you are eating plenty of calcium-rich foods, especially dairy foods, fortified soya products and canned fish with bones.

Eating calcium-rich foods may also help lower your risk of pregnancy-induced hypertension or pre-eclampsia. This can be a risk throughout pregnancy, but might first become apparent during this stage (see also page 239). Your antenatal checks will include measuring your blood pressure to check for this.

Iron supplements

Although some doctors like to recommend iron supplements to all pregnant women, not everyone needs them, and they can cause constipation. If your doctor says that you are anaemic, ask if your plasma ferritin status has been measured. This shows how much stored iron you have and is a more reliable indicator than your haemoglobin level.

If you decide not to take an iron supplement, or you do not need one, it is important that you eat iron-rich foods such as lean red meat, poultry, fortified breakfast cereals and canned sardines and pilchards.

Fibre

Fibre is essential for a healthy digestive system and for preventing constipation. It also helps to keep blood-sugar levels constant. There are two types of fibre, soluble and insoluble, and you need both in your diet. Soluble fibre helps you to feel full for longer and maintains an even release of sugars into the blood. Insoluble fibre prevents constipation by making the transit of food through the body quicker, and carrying away waste products in stools.

Mainly soluble apples, legumes, oats, pears and rye bread

Mainly insoluble beans, fruit, green leafy vegetables, lentils and wholegrain cereals

Weight gain

Starting pregnancy at a healthy weight and gaining weight at a moderate pace is the ideal and will help you to stay healthy. Exactly how much weight you gain depends on several factors, including how many babies you're carrying and your body mass index (BMI) [see page 157] when you became pregnant.

The rate at which you gain weight may vary from week to week. And, unfortunately, little is known about the best time to put on weight in pregnancy. Some research suggests that gaining very little weight early on – when you may be suffering from morning sickness – has less effect on fetal growth than poor weight gain late in the second or third trimester. Some women gain weight very inconsistently, piling on the pounds early and then much less later on. Nothing is necessarily unhealthy about this pattern.

Recommended weight gain

Less than 19 BMI (underweight)	12.5 to 18 kg (28 to 40 lbs)
20 to 26 BMI (normal weight)	11.5 to 16 kg (25 to 35 lbs)
27 to 30 BMI (overweight)	7 to 11.5 kg (15 to 25 lbs)
30 BMI or more (obese)	7 kg (15 lbs) or less

These numbers refer to total weight gain during the entire pregnancy, so you won't know whether you hit the target until delivery day. These recommendations are for women expecting one baby. If you're expecting twins or triplets you may gain considerably more. An average total gain of 15.5 to 20.5 kg (34 to 45 lbs) for twins and 20.5 to 23 kg (45 to 50 lbs) for triplets is likely depending on the length of your pregnancy.

Bear in mind, too, that the recommended weight gains are only a guide: women who gain very little or more than average can still have healthy babies. However, if you are underweight or very overweight, you may be advised to see a nutritionist or dietitian for specific advice on what and how much you should eat.
It's important not to become fanatical about how much you weigh. In the United Kingdom, healthcare providers have stopped routinely weighing women at every antenatal check-up, because it is more effective to check your baby's growth by measuring the fundal height (see page 144) or, if there's cause for concern, by scheduling you for a series of ultrasounds.

Much of the weight you put on during pregnancy will be gone soon after you give birth. Mothers usually lose one-half of their pregnancy weight gain in the first six weeks postpartum

Expecting twins or triplets

Additional calorie needs continue on from the first trimester (see page 99) with a weight gain of 0.7 kg (1.5 lb) a week recommended from now on. Although there are no specific UK recommendations, the US Institute of Medicine advises a daily supplement for women expecting twins or more from the twelfth week. That provides 30 mg iron, 250mg calcium, 15mg zinc, 2mg copper, 2mg vitamin B6, 50mg vitamin C, 50mcg vitamin D and 300 mcg folic acid.

Where most of the weight goes

Baby	39%
Blood	22%
Amniotic fluid	11%
Uterus	1%
Placenta	9%
Breasts	8%

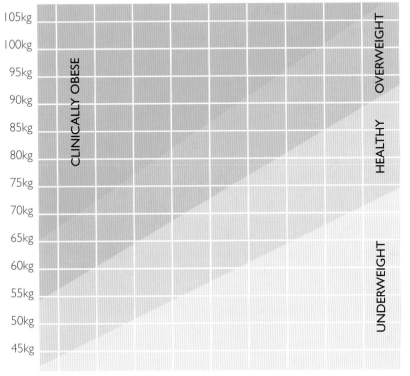

105kg
100kg
95kg
90kg
85kg
80kg
75kg
70kg
65kg
60kg
55kg
50kg
45kg

CLINICALLY OBESE

OVERWEIGHT

HEALTHY

UNDERWEIGHT

150cm 155cm 160cm 165cm 170cm 175cm 180cm 185cm 190cm

BMI Readings

Body mass index is calculated by taking your weight in kilograms (kg) dividing by your height in metres (m) then dividing the result by your height in metres (m) again. The totals equate as follows:

up to 19 = underweight
20-26 = healthy
27 and over = overweight
30 or more = clinically obese

Exercise

During this second trimester, you are in a great stage of pregnancy when you probably feel better than ever; your energy levels should be higher, too.

Providing your pregnancy is progressing well, gentle-to- moderate exercise is highly recommended. Exercise can help relieve many of the symptoms caused by the physical changes to your body such as general aches and pains and constipation and cramps. Aerobic exercise is good for the latter. If you've been exercising in the first trimester, you may feel able to increase the length of each session. Activities like swimming, walking, stationary cycling, t'ai chi and special antenatal aerobics, pilates and yoga are all good choices.

Some guidelines

- Avoid any high-impact activities or bouncy movements
- Don't exercise on your back as your baby's weight can restrict blood flow back to your heart.
- Allow plenty of time when changing positions.
- Avoid standing still too long and take care when standing up if you've been exercising sitting or lying down.

Pelvic floor exercises

As well as doing a good all-over work-out, strengthening your pelvic floor and abdominal muscles can be helpful for a healthy pregnancy and delivery. Your pelvic-floor muscles form a supportive 'hammock' within your pelvis, encircling the urethra, vagina and rectum. Pelvic-floor exercises – also called Kegels after the doctor who introduced them – will help to tone these hard-working muscles, enabling them to support the weight of your growing baby and to help push your baby out during delivery. Also, keeping these muscles toned will enable them to recover more quickly after the birth, so preventing problems such as stress incontinence (see page 220). You can carry out your pelvic-floor exercises literally anywhere – sitting in the car, watching TV, even standing in the checkout queue.

To practise Kegels

1 Identify the correct muscles. Next time you urinate, try to break the flow of urine briefly. Remember how this feels – the muscles that you use to stop the flow are your pelvic-floor muscles. Once you have identified these muscles, don't repeat this exercise during urination. If your bladder isn't emptied completely each time, you may get a urinary tract infection.

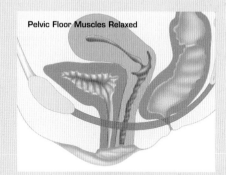

Pelvic Floor Muscles Relaxed

2 Simply tighten your pelvic-floor muscles, hold for a count of five, then slowly release them. You might like to imagine your pelvic floor as an elevator. As it ascends to each floor, try to pull up your muscles a little more until they're completely tight. Then, as the elevator descends floor by floor, gradually relax the muscles until it reaches the ground floor. Repeat five times.

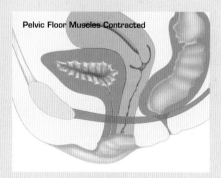

Pelvic Floor Muscles Contracted

3 Repeat the exercise several times a day. Initially, it may seem like hard work even reaching a count of five because these muscles tire easily, but you'll soon be able to build up your repetitions.

Breast care

As soon as you find out that you're pregnant, you may begin to notice that your breasts become fuller and more tender. From about week 16, the nipples and areolae will be noticeably darker, your nipples more prominent and the little glands on the areolae – known as Montgomery's tubercles – enlarge, resembling goose pimples.

These changes are caused by the large amounts of oestrogen and progesterone your body produces during pregnancy. These hormones cause the duct system inside your breasts to grow and branch out, in preparation for milk production and breastfeeding after your baby is born. As your pregnancy advances, the veins on your breasts will become more prominent, stepping up the blood supply to your breasts.

Well-supported breasts

As an expectant mother, it's vitally important to look after your breasts. Breasts themselves contain no muscles and so are supported by the muscles on the chest wall. Unsupported or badly supported breasts are more likely to

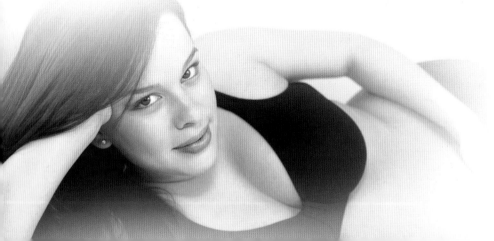

develop stretchmarks (see page 174) or to sag, so even if you have never felt the need for a bra before, you should wear one now.

Check the fit of your existing bras or bra tops, and if they don't offer good support or if they squeeze your breasts in any way, invest in some new, well-fitting ones. By the end of nine months, your breasts may be up to two cup sizes larger than before, and the measurement around your chest, below your breasts, will probably increase as your ribs expand to accommodate your growing baby. After the birth, and once you have stopped breastfeeding, your breasts will reduce in size, but probably won't be the same size and shape as they were before pregnancy.

You won't need special maternity bras for most of your pregnancy, but you should buy a new bra each time your breast size increases so much that you feel uncomfortable and cramped inside your existing one. Some women find they need new bras from around week 8 and most will need a larger size again at about week 36. These bras also will be useful for the first weeks after the birth, so you may want to buy one suitable for breastfeeding. Every woman develops differently, however, so be guided by the changes in your size and shape, not by the calendar. If your breasts become particularly large and heavy, a sleep bra (a lightweight maternity bra worn through the night) may help to make you feel more comfortable.

What to look for in a bra
- **Wide, adjustable shoulder straps** These are more comfortable than narrow straps – which can dig into your skin – because the weight is distributed more evenly.
- **A high proportion of cotton** Natural fibres allow your skin to breathe.
- **A broad band of elastic under the cups** This will support your breasts as they become heavier.
- **An adjustable back** The ideal is to have four hook-and-eye fastenings so that you can loosen your bra as your ribcage expands.
- **No underwiring** The stiff wire can pinch and damage your breast tissues, so go for a softer fit.

Care of the back

A strong back is essential during pregnancy to cope with your larger front load. Strengthening abdominal and buttock muscles and stretching hip flexors, upper back muscles and pectorals will help protect it against long-term problems and help you maintain a good posture. Increased blood flow to the pelvic area, however, softens and relaxes the tissues and ligaments in preparation for labour so they become more flexible and more easily strained. This puts your body off balance, altering your centre of gravity and this is aggravated by the extra weight you are now carrying.

Keep your back in good shape

- Adjust your posture when standing to compensate for the shift in your centre of gravity (see page 193).
- Sit on chairs with good back support. Also, make sure your knees are elevated above your hips.
- Sleep on your side on a firm mattress. Keep a pillow between your legs and under your bump to support your back.
- Lift properly so that you don't strain your back: place your feet shoulder-width apart. Don't bend at the waist but at the knees. As you lift, push up with your thighs and keep your back straight.
- Do not lift or carry heavy objects. But if you do carry bags, make sure the weight is evenly distributed: if you carry groceries in your hands, divide the load into two bags and carry one in each hand; if you carry a small backpack with straps, carry it on both shoulders.
- Wear flat or low-heeled shoes.
- Apply a heated pad to painful areas. Massage also can be very effective.
- If you are carrying larger or multiple babies, wear a support belt – a special belt that fits just below your bump; avoid wearing it all the time, as it can weaken your abdominal muscles.

Shoulder shrug

This can strengthen the trapezius (upper back muscles), which will help to improve your upper body posture.

1 Stand with your feet slightly wider than hip-width and keep your knees soft. Rest your arms by your sides and hold a small weight firmly in each hand, with your palms facing inwards. Tilt your pelvis, tighten the abdominals to lift your baby and stand tall.

2 Lift your shoulders up towards your ears in a shrugging action. Pause briefly at the top, then lower, pressing your shoulders down as far as possible. Keep your elbows soft, your back lifted and your neck long. Then repeat as directed.

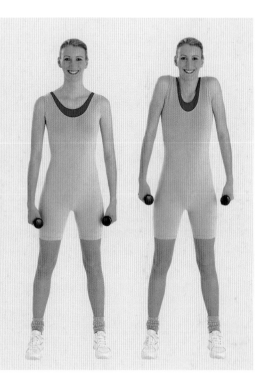

COMBATTING 2ND TRIMESTER SIDE EFFECTS

Now that the fatigue and sickness of the early weeks have worn off, you will probably find that you are feeling a lot better and have more energy to cope with everyday tasks. Nevertheless, you may still experience a few minor problems.

The intestinal muscles also become more relaxed, which can cause complaints such as heartburn (the relaxation of the sphincter muscles at the top of the stomach allows a backflow of acid), and constipation, due to fewer bowel movements. You may find that you need to pass water more often because your baby is pressing down on your bladder. And as your body holds more water when you're pregnant, your fingers, ankles and feet could become swollen, especially if you've been standing for a long time or you are hot (see page 214). There also can be changes to your skin.

Excessive salivation

Overproduction of saliva, which is sometimes called ptyalism, can be a problem but only in the first half of pregnancy. The symptoms include: producing double the amount of bitter-tasting saliva; a thickened tongue and swollen cheeks, caused by enlarged salivary glands. Ptyalism appears to be more common in women who have morning sickness, and it can make the nausea worse temporarily.

What you can do to help
- Cut down on starchy and dairy foods, but still follow a balanced diet (see page 49).
- Eat fruit, as this can ease symptoms.
- Mints, chewing gum, frequent small meals and crackers can help to reduce the amount of saliva produced.
- Try brushing or rinsing your teeth with minty products to freshen your mouth.
- Suck on a piece of lemon or lemon drops.

Forgetfulness and loss of concentration

Forgetfulness accompanied by a loss of concentration during pregnancy is fairly common. It's not something you need to worry about, it isn't a medical problem, and it will resolve in time. Forgetfulness may stem from the stress involved with planning for birth, future parenthood and possibly a move to larger quarters. Some women feel a little overwhelmed by these huge life changes and concerns about the future can crowd the mind of an otherwise clearheaded person. Pregnancy is a wonderfully exciting time, but as your hormones play havoc with your body, it's not surprising you may sometimes find you're not dealing with certain situations as easily as usual. Some women, too, find that anxiety about particular aspects of pregnancy – the health and wellbeing of their baby, for example, results in a lack of concentration on other matters.

Cutting down on your workload by delegating more may help to relieve stress as will socialising less if you are not getting enough sleep – sleep deprivation affects concentration. Take more time for yourself just to sit and relax and, at times, do nothing but think about your baby.

What you can do to help

- Carry a small notebook in which you can jot down reminders or use your computer, mobile phone or PDA alerts.
- Keep a detailed daily calendar.
- Always keep frequently used items, such as keys, in one place.
- Sprinkle a few drops of essential oil of rosemary on a tissue and inhale when you need to stay focused.

Forgetfulness and lack of concentration can cause frustration, so you need to devise strategies that can help you remember what is important.

Slow down

Use this meditation when you want to

- Stop feeling pressured by the burdens of your life

- Slow down, because you're worried stress may be interfering with your thought processes

- Deal with anxiety about a particular aspect of your pregnancy

How to practise this meditation

Regular meditation can give you a sense of inner peace and tranquillity so the things that used to cause you anxiety, stress you no longer. Begin by concentrating on your breathing, feeling your body and mind slowing down as you count each out-breath. Use visualisation to imagine yourself as the calm, controlled person you would like to be.

See yourself in any situation in which you are likely to become stressed. Picture how you would like to deal with that situation, how calm you are, how in control. As you come out of your meditation, keep that image with you, so that the next time you are aware of becoming stressed, it will immediately spring to mind.

mini meditation
Immediate stress buster

If you are feeling particularly tense but can't find the time or privacy to meditate alone for a while, this is a very good temporary stress-buster. Start to be aware of each movement you make. Notice how your body feels, how quick and jerky your actions are, think how you may be hurrying to fit more and more things into an already stressful day.

Then carry on your tasks, but make a concerted effort to do them more slowly. Give yourself time to make each conscious movement. Watch your hands as they type or write or go about your daily chores. Slow your voice down, however much in a hurry you are, when you are speaking. Remember: saving seconds will ultimately succeed only in adding minutes of stress to your life. As your movements ease up, let the thoughts rushing through your head slow down too. Start this again each time you begin to feel tense.

Constipation

Hard and difficult-to-pass stools may be the result of high levels of progesterone, which relax the bowel, meaning that waste matter passes through your system more sluggishly. At the same time, your expanding uterus squashes your intestine. Taking iron supplements can make the problem worse.

Avoiding becoming constipated is far more pleasant than trying to solve the problem, so drink plenty of water (at least 6–8 large glasses a day) and increase the amount of fibre (see page 154) you eat. Keeping active will also help, so try yoga (often there are pregnancy-specific classes), walking or swimming.

What to do to help

- Eat plenty of high-fibre foods such as bran cereals, fruit and vegetables. Some women find it helpful to eat popcorn, but go for the natural kind, without added butter, oil or salt. Too much high-fibre food can cause discomfort, bloating or wind so you may have to experiment to see which foods you tolerate best.
- Drink plenty of fluids – watered-down fruit juice, milk and water are fine. Ginger tea may help.
- Eat prunes or drink a glass of prune juice every day.
- If necessary, take a stool softener. Consider Fybogel or other products containing natural ispaghula husk; these can be bought over the counter. You can take them regularly, once or twice a day. It's best to avoid laxatives, as they can cause abdominal cramping and, occasionally, uterine contractions.
- Exercise regularly. It encourages the bowels to become more active and promotes daily bowel movements.

Heartburn

A burning sensation, which occurs in the upper part of your abdomen, near the breastbone, is very common in the latter part of pregnancy. It's the result of acids produced in the stomach being pushed up into the tube connecting your mouth to your stomach.

Heartburn is more pronounced during pregnancy for two reasons. The high level of progesterone that your body is producing can slow digestion and relax the sphincter muscle between the oesophagus and the stomach, which normally prevents the upward movement of stomach acids.

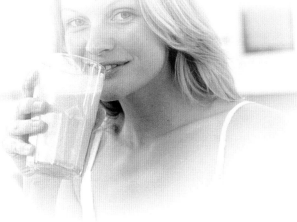

What you can do to help

- Eat small, frequent meals.
- Drink milk to help neutralise stomach acid.
- Take a safe-for pregnancy antacid after meals and at bedtime.
- Munch on dry cream crackers when you feel heartburn. They may neutralize the pain.
- Avoid spicy, fatty and greasy food and fizzy drinks.
- Avoid lying down after a meal and eating just before bedtime – heartburn occurs most readily when you lie down.
- Wear loose clothes.
- Try sleeping with your head elevated on several pillows.

Wind and bloating

Burping and passing wind at inopportune times can be highly embarrassing but are inescapable complaints in pregnancy. Even before the end of the first trimester, you may find that your belly looks bloated and distended – an unwelcome side effect of the hormone progesterone, which causes you to retain water. This hormone slows down the bowels also, causing them to enlarge. Oestrogen, the other key pregnancy hormone, causes your uterus to enlarge, which also makes your tummy feel bigger.

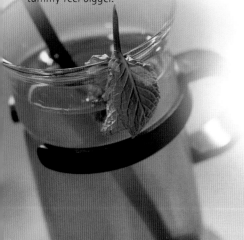

What you can do to help

- There's very little you can do to prevent burping or passing wind, but try to avoid becoming constipated (see page 168), because that may make things worse.
- Avoid eating large meals, which may leave you feeling bloated and uncomfortable, or foods you know make the problem even worse. These vary from person to person, but some common offenders include onions, cabbage, fried foods, rich sauces and beans.
- Don't rush your meals. This can cause you to swallow air, which can form painful pockets of air in your gut.
- Drinking peppermint or camomile tea may be helpful.

Leg problems

Aching legs

As pregnancy progresses, your legs and feet have to support more weight and aches and pains become quite common. These can be made more miserable when retained moisture makes your feet puffy, too (see also page 214).

What you can do to help

- Wear flat shoes for everyday. You might find that support sandals (such as Birkenstock), which can be worn with socks in the winter or trainers produce the best results.
- Use a foot moisturiser or massage oil morning and night on aching parts.
- Try a foot bath into which you add two drops essential oil of orange or petitgrain and submerge your legs for up to 20 minutes.

Cramping

Often worse when you've gone to bed, cramp occurs more frequently and painfully as pregnancy progresses. No one's sure exactly what causes cramp – one theory links it to low levels of magnesium or calcium. Fatigue and a build-up of fluid in the legs at the end of the day are also thought to be contributing factors. Some doctors believe that cramp in your legs may be related to a decrease in circulation, which gets worse when you're sitting down.

What you can do to help

- Walking about in bare feet can help to ease the pain of cramp.
- Stretching and extending your legs and feet should help to diminish the pain of cramp.
- Leg massage may help to minimise the pain.

Round ligament pain

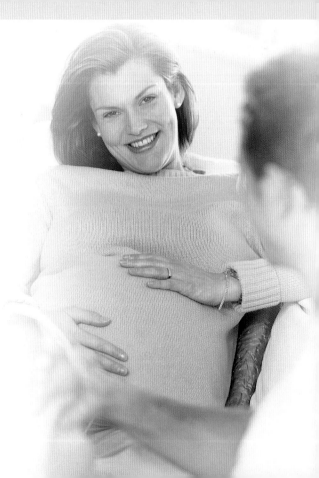

Between 18 and 24 weeks, you may feel a sharp pain or a dull ache on one or both sides of your lower abdomen or near your groin. It's often stronger when you move quickly or stand, and it may fade if you lie down. The round ligaments are bands of fibrous tissue on each side of the uterus that attach it to the labia. As the uterus enlarges in the second trimester, the stretching of these ligaments may cause discomfort. While it can be quite uncomfortable, it's perfectly normal. The good news is that it usually goes away, or at least decreases considerably, after 24 weeks.

What you can do to help
- Take breaks from standing or walking, and put your feet up when sitting.
- Always mention any abdominal pain when you have an antenatal check-up so that you can be reassured that there is nothing wrong.

Skin problems

Overall, you may find that your skin becomes softer, due to its increased ability to retain moisture, and that you have the characteristic 'glow' of pregnancy, which is partly due to an increase in hormone levels. However, you may notice other changes to your skin. Pregnant women, for example, often perspire more as a result of the action of pregnancy hormones on sweat glands all over the body; for this reason, heat rashes are more common. Most skin changes go away in the first six months after the birth, but some may remain permanently.

Hormones make your skin more susceptible to the effects of the sun, so make sure you use sufficient sun protection strategies (see page 199).

Chloasma

The skin around your cheeks, nose and eyes may also darken. This is called chloasma or 'the mask of pregnancy' and appears dark in fair-skinned women and light in dark-skinned women. Chloasma is due to hormonal influences on skin pigment cells. Exposure to the sun can make these changes darker.

Linea nigra

You may notice a dark line running from your pubic bone up to your navel. Called the linea nigra, this is usually more prominent in darker-skinned women.

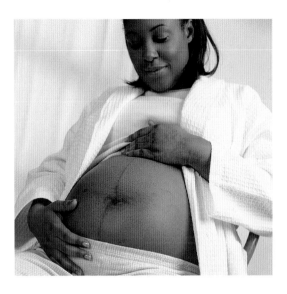

Acne

Some women who suffer from acne find that their skin improves during pregnancy. Others find that the condition becomes worse, and women who do not normally have acne may develop it or be subject to spots. You may be able to help to control spots by cutting down on fats in your diet and exercising regularly. Always consult your healthcare provider before taking any acne medication, as it may contain chemicals that could affect your baby. Acne and spots usually clear up in the second trimester.

Skin tags, moles and freckles

Minuscule tags of skin are also a common occurrence in high-friction areas, although it isn't totally clear why they occur. It's not a good idea to rush to the dermatologist to have them removed. Existing moles, freckles or skin blemishes may become darker. If a new mole appears or an existing one changes appreciably in size or appearance, see your doctor.

Stretchmarks

Deep pinky-red streaks occur when the collagen protein fibres that usually give the skin support are broken down by the effect of pregnancy hormones. They affect three in five women and are most likely to appear on the stomach, the sides of the breasts and the thighs. They fade to silvery grey or white several months after pregnancy. You are more likely to get stretch marks if your mother had them.

There's no completely effective way to prevent stretchmarks, and no cream is available that will get rid of them entirely, but there are things you can do to help prevent or soften their appearance.

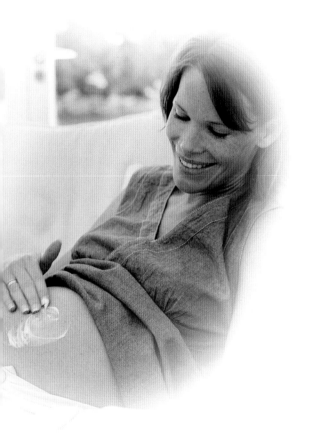

What you can do to help

- Eat sensibly and avoid gaining too much weight. If you gain a great deal of weight in a short space of time, your skin won't have a chance to adapt and will have to stretch to accommodate your new shape.
- Wear a well-fitting bra throughout your pregnancy. Keep your growing breasts adequately supported as they become heavier.
- Wear a sleep bra if your breasts are large. Looking after your breasts during the day isn't enough – they need 24-hour care.
- Keep your skin supple and itch-free. Massage cream into your breasts and tummy to elasticize the skin. Cocoa butter or almond oil extract – available from pharmacists – have proved effective for some women. Try a morning and evening massage.

Beat minor ailments

Use this meditation when you want to

- Think positively about your body's reaction to pregnancy

- Try to prevent problems from occurring

- Deal calmly with physical complaints if they do arise

How to practise this meditation

As you get bigger, you may find it difficult to sit comfortably in one position for any length of time. Don't prevent yourself from shifting as the discomfort could become distracting, but when you do move, try to change positions with the minimum of effort, making sure you have plenty of support and cushions.

To help you immediately refocus, concentrate on your breath and use the same hand position every time as a 'memory cue' to draw you back to where you left off. A common hand position for meditation is with the thumb and forefinger of each hand lightly touching and the other fingers either extended or curled; alternatively, rest your hands on your knees, with your palms turned upwards.

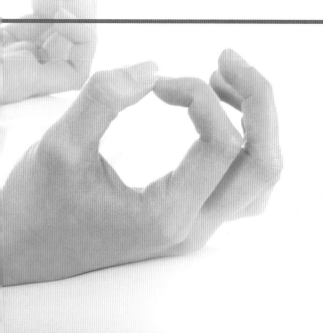

Once you are comfortable and breathing slowly, concentrate on the area of your body you wish to help. For instance, if you are suffering from backache, focus on your back, moving to each point which hurts or feels tense, such as your shoulders or lower back. At each point, as you concentrate on your breaths, imagine the trouble spot feeling flexible, strong and healthy. Spend five to ten breaths on each area, sensing the aches and tension fall away as you do. If you can't pinpoint exactly where the pain is coming from, just visualise your back as a whole. Be aware of particular times or situations when you tend to become strained, and mentally remind yourself to use this bodyscan technique to minimise any problems.

Keeping in touch with your unborn baby

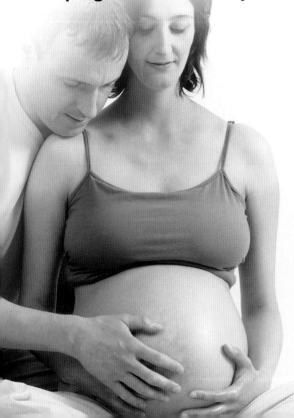

Being aware of your unborn baby is the first step to bonding, creating a closeness that will last you a lifetime. It will also help you adjust to the idea of parenthood, and help make your pregnancy a more rewarding one.

Your baby is not, as was once thought, a fetus without a personality or feelings whose senses only awaken once born. On the contrary, studies have indicated that babies are aware of and can react to stimuli from outside the uterus long before birth. From the first few weeks after conception your baby could brush the inside of your uterus and by now can consciously move in response to external stimuli, such as the stroke of your hand. By sixteen weeks, the ears have developed enough for sounds to be heard – your reassuring heartbeat, the sound of your voice and the rumblings of your stomach – and by twenty-four weeks more distant sounds such as music and your partner's voice can be heard. At the end of this trimester, the eyelids will have separated and your baby will be able to make out changes in brightness for the first time, shying away if a light is too fierce.

Your baby will be very much in tune with your own feelings from the second trimester of pregnancy onward. When you experience different emotions, chemicals are released into your bloodstream and cross the placenta to your baby – excitement and laughter release endorphins, for example, which help your body respond to stress and will also give your baby that 'feelgood' factor, too; while anger or stress releases adrenaline (see overleaf) and will thus make your body feel tense to your baby.

By being aware of your baby, you can tune in to his or her likes and dislikes. For instance, notice if your baby moves more when you play a certain piece of music, or whether his or her activity increases when you are relaxing in a warm bath, the water gently swaying and washing over you. Here are some practical tips for getting close to that little person inside you.

What you should do

- Touch and stroke your baby as often as possible. The movement and warmth of your hand is very reassuring.
- Talk and sing aloud to your baby. Experiments have shown that, once born, babies can recognise words and music they heard when they were in the uterus.
- Try to direct your thoughts towards your baby. Think positively, say what you feel, explore your expectations and don't worry about the odd negative thought – it won't have an adverse effect.
- Your baby will respond to your movements, being lulled by gentle swaying or walking, and becoming agitated if you are dashing around. So keep your actions relaxed and calm.

Bond with your baby

Use this meditation when you want to

- Feel close to your baby

- Tune in to your baby's movements

- Let your baby know how much love you have to give

How to practise this meditation

This technique involves playing different types of music to see whether you get a response from your baby. Some mothers have found their babies respond to the eerie high and low frequencies of whale and dolphin sounds; others have found vocal or choral music most effective (probably because this is closest in pitch and tone to the mother's voice).

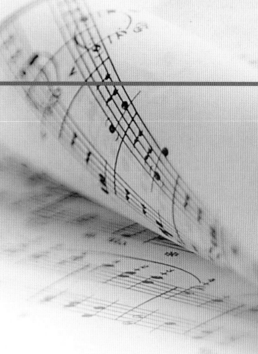

Sit or lie in any position that feels comfortable. As you let the music wash over you, concentrate on your breathing, still your mind and let your body relax. Be aware that your baby can not only hear the music but will also sense the slowing down of your own actions and the tension leaving you. You may want to visualise your baby lying in the uterus, cradled in the warm fluid of the amniotic sac and being soothed by the peace surrounding you. Or you could chant a mantra, so that the sounds reverberate through your body to your baby: choose a word that encapsulates the closeness you feel to your unborn child.

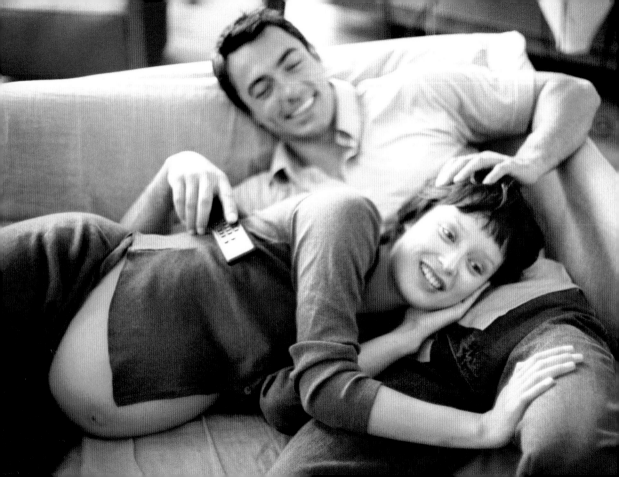

Chapter 4

The third trimester

THE FINAL MONTHS

You may feel like your pregnancy has been going on forever, but now that you're in the third trimester, an end to the long months of waiting is in sight and it won't be long before you'll have the thrilling experience of holding your baby at last.

The larger you get during these weeks, the more difficult it will become to carry out tasks you found simple earlier in your pregnancy, such as shopping,

cleaning the house, even getting out of the bath! You will tire more easily, so take things easy, napping when you can. It is important to relax in order to cope with any problems or anxieties that occur as you near your labour, so you're well prepared for the incredible event of the birth of your child.

Antenatal care

From the beginning of your third trimester, you will be offered an antenatal check at least every two weeks until week 36 and then every week from week 36 until you deliver. During these visits your blood pressure will be measured and your urine checked for protein and possibly glucose. Your baby's size and position will be measured and his heartbeat monitored. Your rhesus status (see page 122) will be tested and at week 28, you will be given a blood test for anaemia.

If your blood pressure rises or your urine test is positive for the presence of protein, your healthcare provider will refer you for further tests to rule out the presence of pre-eclampsia (see page 239). You may have certain blood tests to check for blood abnormalities that can occur with pre-eclampsia, such as low platelets and abnormal liver function tests.

Group B streptococcus test
Approximately 10 per cent of pregnant women carry in their vaginas a bacteria that can cause a severe bacterial infection in newborn babies. Known as Strep B, it can be treated with antibiotics during delivery if you have tested positive. Many practitioners, therefore, test for this in the late stages of pregnancy.

Checking on baby
Usually, in the last few weeks, your baby will take up a head-down position. If you baby is not in the head-down position at 36 weeks, however, your healthcare provider may advise steps to try to turn your baby around into the correct position so that you can have a normal delivery. Performing a simple meditation has proved effective (see page 259), so, too, has assuming a breech tilt position. If these don't work, your doctor may perform an external version.

Breech tilt
Lie on your back with your knees flexed and place four plump pillows or cushions under your buttocks so that your pelvis is higher than your stomach. Alternatively, kneel down on the floor with your buttocks raised as high as possible while your head rests on your folded arms. Remain in the position for a minimum of 10 minutes twice a day.

Date/Time	Place	Procedure

Head down

This is the best position for birth, and more than 95 per cent of babies naturally adopt it before labour. If your baby's back is facing your abdomen, this is called occiput anterior; if her back is turned towards your spine, this is called occiput posterior. This position can cause severe backache during labour.

Breech presentation

As many as 4 per cent of babies settle bottom or feet first. This is known as a breech presentation. There are small, but significant, risks to the vaginal birth of a breech baby, especially for first babies, and some doctors will only deliver breech babies by Caesarean. However, you can carry out exercises to move the baby into a head-down position.

Transverse lie

Less than 1 per cent of babies are positioned across the uterus. This is known as a transverse or oblique lie, and it makes a normal vaginal birth impossible. It is sometimes possible to change these positions using the breech tilt after 32 weeks and external version at 37-38 weeks.

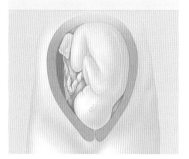
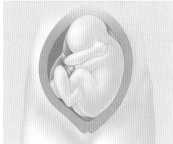
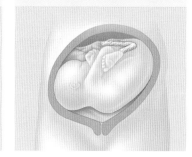

External version

When there's enough amniotic fluid to allow for a small amount of movement, your obstetrician may manipulate your abdomen to encourage your baby to slowly turn. This procedure is not without risks, which your obstetrician should discuss with you. Success rates vary from 50 to 70 per cent.

Kick chart

Your baby's movements should increase and be easier to keep track of now. After 28 weeks, you should be able to count at least ten movements every day, between 9 a.m. and 9 p.m. It's a good idea to record them on a chart and to advise your healthcare provider immediately if you become aware of a significant decrease.

SAMPLE KICK-COUNT SHEET														
	WEEK 39							WEEK 40						
TIME	M	T	W	T	F	S	S	M	T	W	T	F	S	S
9 am														
9.30 am														
10 am														
10.30 am														
11 am														
11.30 am														
12 pm														
12.30 pm														
1 pm														
1.30 pm														
2 pm														
2.30 pm														
3 pm														
3.30 pm														
4 pm														
4.30 pm														
5 pm														
5.30 pm														
6 pm														
6.30 pm														
7 pm														
7.30 pm														
8 pm														
8.30 pm														
9 pm														
If less than ten movements by 9 pm, record total number here														
9														
8														
7														
6														
5														
4														
3														
2														
1														

Healthy eating

If you are a first-time mother, during the next few weeks your baby's head will engage, and this should help release some of the pressure you have been feeling on your stomach and internal organs. Until this happens, you may find that you would rather eat small meals and snacks than full-size meals. Try having one or two portions of a main course and eating some vegetables or a salad or dessert later on.

Your baby is now fully developed and will be building up her fat deposits, ready for the outside world. You need to continue to eat well, even if you can manage only small portions. A varied diet, rich in fruit and vegetables, will help to further develop your baby's immune system.

Around this time, many mums-to-be find that their digestive systems slow down and they experience constipation. This is caused by a combination of factors: your baby is exerting considerable pressure by lying on your intestines; and hormonal changes and a less active lifestyle have a negative effect. Prevention is far better than cure, so if you start to feel any discomfort, increase the amount of water and fibre in

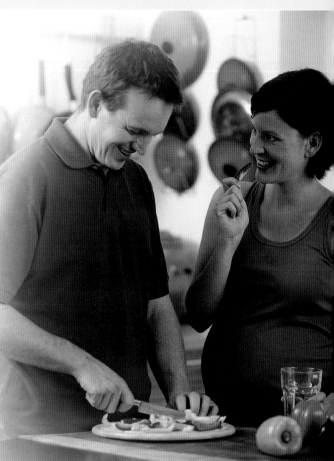

your diet (see also page 154). As the baby is exerting pressure on your bladder, drinking more may not seem an attractive prospect, but water is essential to bulk out the fibre in your stools. Tea and coffee are not the solution – in fact, they can have the opposite effect.

Omega 3 fatty acids

Unsaturated fatty acids are needed at all stages of life, but some are especially important during pregnancy. The omega 3 fatty acids, DHA and EPA, help the development of your baby's eyes, brain, blood and nervous system. These are needed especially during the last trimester when your baby's brain is growing rapidly. If your baby is born prematurely or is of a low birth weight, she can miss out on this important phase, so you will be advised to keep up your supply of these essential nutrients when breastfeeding or if you are bottle feeding, be prescribed a supplemented infant formula for your baby.

Try to include the following in your diet regularly: Oily fish such as salmon, mackerel or herring; nuts and seeds such as sunflower, almonds, etc.; green leafy vegetables; and oil or spreads made from seeds such as sunflower, linseed or rapeseed.

Vitamin B12

At this stage in your pregnancy, your baby's nerves are beginning to develop a protective myelin sheath. This continues after he is born, and is reliant on vitamin B12, which is found almost exclusively in animal products. Ensure that you eat some lean red meat or poultry regularly and have plenty of low-fat dairy products. If you are vegetarian, you will need to take a vitamin supplement and eat fortified breakfast cereals to make sure you are getting enough B12.

Vitamin K

Vital for blood clotting, you should aim to ensure you have sufficient in preparation for childbirth by eating green leafy vegetables such as broccoli, Brussels sprouts, kale and spinach; canteloupe melon; and fortified breakfast cereals, wholemeal bread and pasta.

Exercise

If you feel up to it and have plenty of energy, then continue to exercise although you may prefer to reduce your exercise intensity to a lower level. Omit any movements you find difficult. If you feel tired, try performing just some warming up and stretching exercises; these will help to keep you mobile and reduce muscular and joint stiffness. Avoid standing for long periods and ensure that you allow yourself sufficient time to rest and relax. Your baby's size and weight will increase considerably during these last three months, making your back even more vulnerable.

Pelvic floor exercises

At around 28 weeks start building up the intensity of your pelvic-floor exercises (see page 158). Start to hold each squeeze for a count of 10, and repeat four to six times, at least three times a day.

Vary your technique. Try changing the speed you do the pull ups in order to acquire greater flexibility and control. Count quickly to 10 or 20, alternately contracting and relaxing your pelvic floor each time you say a number. Or, do it slowly, contracting for a slow count of four, waiting for a count of 10 and then slowly releasing the muscles for a count of four.

Remember, you can perform these exercises lying, standing, or sitting without it being visible to anyone else, so try to do them as often as possible – at work, in the car, or watching television. Do not, however, perform them while you are urinating as this may cause infection.

Take care when exercising

- Remember to tilt your pelvis and tighten your abdominals at all times, and take care when moving from one position to another.
- Keep your movements controlled and avoid rushing exercises; a few selected exercises performed correctly will be more beneficial than a larger programme done badly.

Strengthening your pelvic floor

1 **Slow contractions** Stand, lie or sit with your feet slightly apart. Draw up and tighten the muscles around the anal sphincter; then hold. Slowly tighten the muscles around the urinary sphincter as well and lift up through the vagina. Hold for a count of 6, release with control, then repeat as recommended above right. If you've never worked these muscles, it may be difficult to isolate the movements individually, but it will get easier with practice.

2 **Fast contractions** Stand, lie or sit with your feet slightly apart. Tighten all your pelvic floor muscles in one contraction. Hold for a count of 1, then release slowly and with control. Continue as directed above.

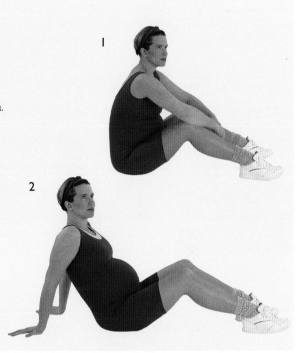

Back care

During the last trimester particularly, as your abdomen enlarges and your baby becomes heavier, there is a forward shift in your centre of gravity, which can result in bad posture, upper back and shoulder pain and lower back discomfort. You may find yourself leaning backwards or stooping forwards to adjust your centre of gravity. This can strain the muscles around your spine, resulting in backache. Hormones released during pregnancy result in softened and stretched ligaments, which also make your back more vulnerable to strains. Maintaining good posture in your everyday activities may help to eliminate these stresses and strains. Initially, you'll find that you have to make a conscious effort to correct and keep a balanced posture, but after a while you'll find it more natural. Core stability exercises such as Pilates can help greatly with posture and back pain in pregnancy.

Finding a good posture

Check that your weight is evenly distributed between your feet. Stand tall and lengthen your neck – it can help to imagine a string pulling you up through the top of your head. Try to look straight ahead and keep your chin parallel to the floor.

Relax your shoulders. If you find that your shoulders are slumping forwards, push your shoulder blades together until you find a comfortable – but not rigid – position. This will help to open out your chest.

To keep your lower back strong and to support your baby, tighten your abdominals. Once you have found a comfortable position, try to maintain it. Never adopt the two extremes of pushing your pelvis all the way forwards or all the way backwards. A common mistake many pregnant women make is to let the weight of their bump pull their spine forwards, which puts strain on the lower back.

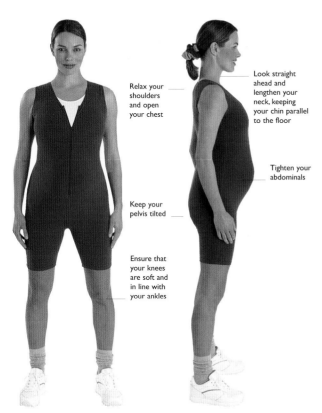

Relax your shoulders and open your chest

Look straight ahead and lengthen your neck, keeping your chin parallel to the floor

Tighten your abdominals

Keep your pelvis tilted

Ensure that your knees are soft and in line with your ankles

Stand tall

Drop your shoulders so that they are relaxed. Tuck in your buttocks and straighten up your back. Lengthen your neck and raise your head as though the centre at the top is being pulled towards the ceiling. Avoid tensing up your knees and keep your weight evenly spread between your toes and heels. When you are ironing or washing dishes, avoid hunching over the board or sink. If you have a low sink, put a large washing-up bowl on top of the sink and do the dishes in the bowl. Lower the ironing board and sit on a stool so that you are ironing at waist height.

Sit straight

Whether you are sitting in a chair or on the floor, always keep your back straight. When you sit in a chair, sit flush against the back of the chair so that it supports the small of your back. If your chair doesn't provide this support comfortably, you can place a small cushion or rolled-up towel in the small of your back. Keep your legs uncrossed to prevent poor circulation.

Getting up in stages

For safety sake, raise yourself from a lying position in a series of stages.

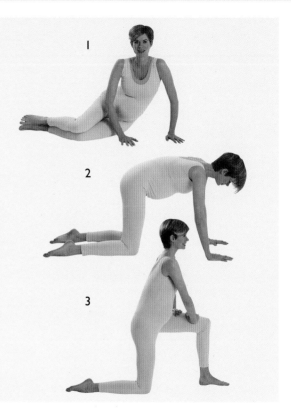

1 Bring your knees and feet together and place your hands on the floor to one side of your body. With your elbows soft, roll yourself over into a side kneeling position.

2 Continue to roll over until you are kneeling on your hands and knees. Walk your hands in and slowly bring yourself up into an upright kneeling position, tilting your pelvis as you straighten up.

3 Lift one knee up and place the foot flat on the floor; your knee should be over your ankle. Place both hands on your thigh, tighten your abdominal and buttock muscles and push yourself up to a standing position. Tilt your pelvis and stand tall.

Lie down slowly

Always lie down from a sitting position. When you are seated, slowly swing your legs over the bed or couch so that they are parallel with your hips. Gently lower yourself onto your elbows, so they are supporting your upper body weight. Using your hands, slide down to a lying position.

Easing discomfort

Massage can help to ease backache. As backache also can occur during labour, getting your partner to massage you now will familiarise him with techniques that may help later on. Spend at least 10 minutes on each session.

Kneel on a bed or the floor and relax into a large pile of pillows so that your bump and head are comfortably supported. Place a pillow between your calves and bottom to assist with your circulation.

Placing the flat of his left hand on your left shoulder, your massage partner strokes firmly and slowly down the side of your spine to your buttocks. Before removing his hand, he places his right hand on your shoulder and strokes firmly down again. Then, starting with his right hand on your right shoulder, he should stroke down that side of your spine. He should

continue to alternate between each side. Tell him if the pressure is right.

Next, he uses his thumbs to make small circles in the grooves on either side of your spine, gradually working down, vertebra to vertebra. At the bottom of your back, he makes larger circles using his palms to circle down over your hips.

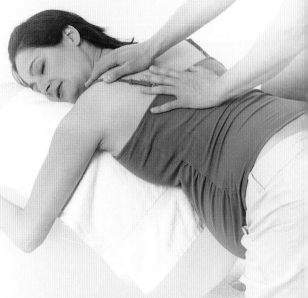

Hand and foot care

You may find that your fingernails split and break more easily during pregnancy; if so, keep them short and wear rubber gloves for washing up and doing housework. You also should use gloves to protect your hands when you're working in the garden and to avoid picking up soil-borne infections (see page 69). Apply hand cream regularly, ideally the type with nail strengthener.

Pregnancy places additional strain on your feet, both through the extra weight they have to bear and through potential swelling (see page 214). You may find that it helps to soak your feet in a bowl of water in the evening and to massage with peppermint foot cream after a bath or shower.

Keep toenails short, but not so short that they may ingrow, and cut them straight across. If you can't reach your toes in the later stages of pregnancy, you may need to ask for some help or have a professional pedicure. It makes sense to go to a reputable beauty salon where the equipment is properly cleaned.

Hand massage

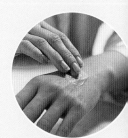

1 Pick up a little cream with the fingers of your right hand. Apply to the back of your left hand using smooth strokes from your fingertips up to your wrist.

2 Turn your left hand over. Cupping it with your right fingers, circle your palm with your right thumb. Apply more cream as needed as you stretch out the palm. Briefly press the centre of your palm to promote relaxation.

3 Turn your left hand back over. Starting at your little finger, circle each knuckle with your right thumb. Slide down each of your fingers with your right thumb and forefinger. When you get to the fingertips, briefly squeeze to stimulate the brain and promote clear thinking.

4 Repeat steps 1-3 using your left hand to apply cream to your right. Interlink fingers and rub your palms together. Flex your fingers and shake your hands.

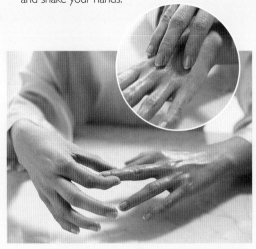

Easing common discomforts

By the third trimester, the ankles often swell, a sign that you need to stop standing for too long, wear comfortable shoes and put your feet up as often as possible. Regularly rotating each foot one way and then the other can help prevent swelling. Other things to ease the problem include massaging the feet with smooth, gentle strokes up the calf and shin from ankle to knee. To a tepid water footbath, add two drops essential oil of bergamot and relax for up to 20 minutes. For hot, swollen feet make it a cool water footbath and add two drops essential oil of grapefruit. If you're really perspiring, throw in a few ice cubes. For itchy (or dry) feet, add two teaspoons jojoba to the water, swishing well to disperse.

Your palms and sometimes the soles of your feet may become red and itchy. Known as palmar erythema, this is caused by increased levels of oestrogen. If your skin is itching unbearably, make sure you see your healthcare provider, as this could be a symptom of cholestasis, a serious liver problem. Asian women are most at risk.

LOOKING AFTER YOUR SKIN, HAIR AND TEETH

Pregnancy can involve a radiant complexion and lustrous hair but it also can encompass less desirable changes. You can help to ameliorate any negative effects by taking proper care of yourself and your changing body. Beauty products targeted specifically at pregnant women don't contain any magic ingredients, despite what they may claim, so use them only if you're really impressed with their results. Thorough, consistent daily routines, however, will keep you looking your best.

Facial skin care

The greater volume of blood circulating in your body combined with the slight rise in body temperature, may give your skin the characteristic pregnancy 'glow' and a soft, velvety texture as it plumps out and retains more moisture. Don't be surprised, however, if your skin becomes a bit unpredictable – unusually dry or greasy, with spots or spider angiomas (tiny broken blood vessels) on your cheeks. Most marks will fade after delivery and your skin type will return to normal, but if you wish to even out your skin colour, use concealer not lightening fluid, which can damage skin.

Daily routine
Cleanse your face at least once a day using a non-soap product suitable for your current skin type. Soap can be too harsh for your face and strip your skin of its natural oils. Adapt your daily skincare routine to accommodate any changes to your complexion and be prepared to keep making minor adjustments as your pregnancy progresses; if you develop spots, scrupulous attention to hygiene is even more important, to keep the pores clear. To tone greasy skin and clean out clogged pores, use a mild astringent but if your skin is

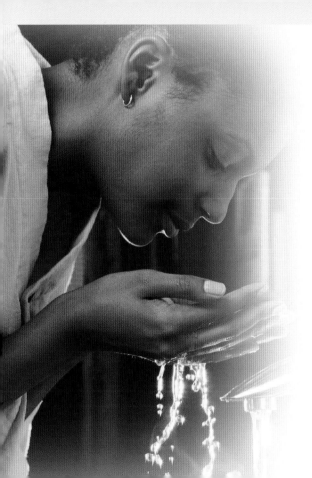

dry, lavish moisturiser on it Allow the moisturiser to sink in and rehydrate your complexion. If your skin becomes dry only in patches, treat it like combination skin: apply more moisturiser to the drier areas.

Facials

If you have regular facials as part of your skin-care routine there's no reason to stop while pregnant. And they are a great way to relax. Facials won't worsen any pregnancy-related skin changes, but your skin may be more sensitive than usual, so always check that any products being used are suitable.

Sun protection

Hormones make your skin more susceptible to the effects of the sun, so that it may burn much more quickly than before. Apply a foundation or moisturising cream containing sunscreen daily, and cover all exposed skin with sun cream with a sun protection factor (SPF) of at least 15 before you leave the house. Don't forget to take care of your lips, too. They may seem drier than usual, so use a moisturising lip balm regularly – on its own or under lipstick – to stop them from cracking.

Body care

Your increased blood flow will probably make you feel warmer than usual and, as a result, you'll sweat more easily than you usually do. Make time for a daily, or even twice daily, bath or shower – use warm water rather than hot, as hot water will open your pores and make you even more likely to sweat. If your skin is feeling dry, a light aqueous cream can be used as a soap substitute or as a moisturising skin cream, which should be applied after washing, while your skin is still wet.

You also can help to prevent sweating by choosing cotton rather than synthetic underwear, and if you wear tights, opt for types with cotton-lined gussets. Wear clothes made of natural rather than synthetic fibres to help you to stay cooler.

Hair removal

Bikini, leg or facial waxes, are topical preparations that contain no substances harmful to a developing baby, so there's no reason why you can't have waxing done during pregnancy. Although there is no known risk of depilatories or bleach harming the baby, your skin may not react well to them, and there is a possibility that

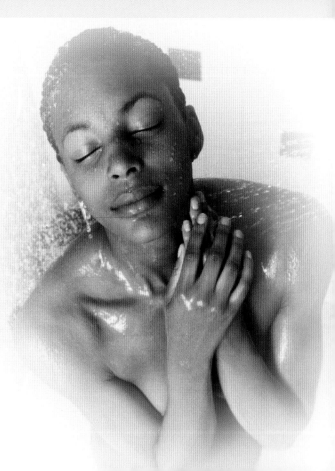

their chemicals can get into the bloodstream. Electrolysis is also not recommended, even though there is no proof that it could harm the baby. Threading, shaving and plucking unwanted hair are safer alternatives.

Abdomen and breasts

The skin over your abdomen and breasts is being stretched considerably and, as a result, may feel particularly dry and itchy. Massage your tummy with a moisturizing cream or oil – a nice way to communicate with your developing baby as well as supplying a well-earned period of relaxation. If your breasts are dry, apply moisturiser here, also. However, avoid over-moisturising your nipples – if they become too soft and damp they may feel sore. If you do experience any discomfort from sore nipples, expose your breasts to the air occasionally while you're relaxing at home.

The breasts of women with silicone or saline breast implants may be affected by pregnancy. Some women have increased breast tenderness as their own breast tissue grows, and that growth combined with the increased size present from the implants stretches the overlying skin to an uncomfortable degree.

If you have flat or inverted nipples and are planning to breastfeed, you may benefit from breast shells, which can help your nipples to protrude and enable your baby to latch on properly. Before your baby is born, it is a good idea to practise putting them on and wearing them underneath your bra.

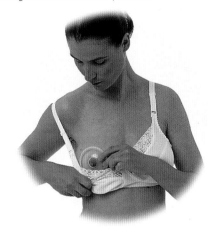

Treating minor skin problems

Irritated skin

When it stretches tight and thins because of hormone changes, skin can become irritated and break out in rashes or even eczema.

What you can do to help

- Avoid biological washing powders, and switch to 'green' home products and DIY materials (If chlorine-treated swimming pools affect you, look for an ozone-treated alternative.)
- Liquidise half a cucumber and apply over the skin as a mask (avoiding the eyes — place refrigerated slices over them). Rest for 10-20 minutes before wiping away and splashing with cool water.
- To a tepid bath, add six drops essential oil of frankincense and swish to disperse just before stepping in.

Dry, flaky skin

If you suffer from eczema or dry skin, this can be exacerbated by pregnancy. If you've previously been prescribed a cortisone cream, check with your doctor that it is safe to use in pregnancy. Instead of soap to wash your face, use a mild, soapless cleanser. Also, make sure you apply your moisturizer while your skin is still damp.

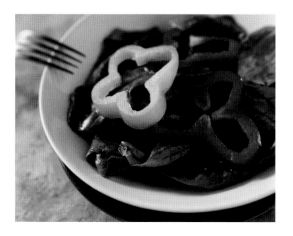

What you can do to help

- Eat foods rich in essential fatty acids – nuts, seeds, small oily fish; vitamin A – red, yellow, orange and dark green fruit and vegetables. eggs, cheese and butter. Also eat foods containing vitamin B5 – meat, fish, wholegrains, pulses and nuts.
- Try a massage cure. Into a base of five teaspoons apricot kernel oil and one teaspoon jojoba, blend one drop each essential oils of sandalwood (to moisturise), neroli (to rebalance sebum production) and patchouli (to heal cracked skin).
- Tone face and neck with a tea made of one bag lime blossom (tillieul) in a mug of boiling water allowed to steep for 20 minutes and applied with a cotton ball soaked in the mixture.

Breakouts and acne

Pregnancy hormones are responsible for increasing (even overproducing) levels of sebum in the skin, which can cause pores to become blocked with shed cells, attracting bacteria and leading to inflammation. Never squeeze or pick! Try to relax (see page 226) – acne is worsened by stress. If you are using an anti-acne medication, make sure that it is safe for pregnancy – some common preparations can be harmful.

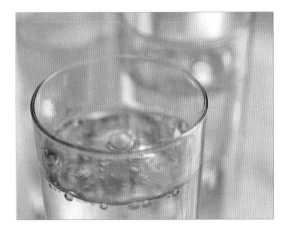

What you can do to help

- Fill up on good sources of vitamin B3 – dairy products, oily fish and chicken, nuts, yeast extract and cereals and cut back on fried, fatty, sugary foods.
- Drink plenty of water to help flush out the waste products the body now finds harder to process.
- After cleansing, soak a cotton ball in rosewater or orange blossom water and wipe the affected area. Dab on a little manuka honey, a potent antibacterial and renowned zit-zapper that acts on bacterial growth and soothes without drying the skin.
- Smooth witch hazel gel over the affected area.
- Use 'noncomedogenic' skin-care products and make-up; these won't clog pores.
- Wash your face frequently using a gentle cleanser; apply an oil-free moisturiser.

Itchy skin

When skin is stretched tight across your belly, the urge to itch can disturb your sleep and may be debilitating. If, after 28 weeks, itching is very intense, consult your healthcare provider. This may be obstetric cholestasis, a medical emergency.

Thread veins

Tiny red veins or clusters of dots on the cheeks and shins may appear worse in pregnancy as blood vessels dilate and constrict more rapidly than usual, making them extra sensitive.

What you can do to help

- Soothe skin by rubbing in handfuls of organic olive oil after a bedtime bath while your skin is still damp.
- Take an oatmeal or rich oil bath; soothe irritated skin by rubbing with an oatmeal bag containing 12 tbsp each oatmeal and powdered milk.
- Fill up on foods rich in vitamin B6 such as bananas, whole grains, peas and beans.
* Use olive oil for cooking and drink plenty of water.

What you can do to help

- Make a toner from a vascular-constrictor herb: pour boiling water over one bag of camomile or marigold tea in a mug and steep for five minutes. Allow to cool, then soak a cotton ball in the mixture and use to apply to the area.
- Massage an oil made of one tsp peach kernel oil, and one drop each essential oils of neroli and sandalwood gently over the affected area.
- Cover up in very hot, humid climes and in cold, windy places, too, to prevent weather damage.

Hair care

Your increased metabolism and boosted circulation may mean that your hair grows faster, while hair loss slows down. This vigorous growth means that your hair will look thicker and more lustrous than usual. Some pregnant women, however, are less lucky and find that their hair becomes greasy or unusually dry or lifeless. Don't worry if this happens to you: any changes that you experience will be short-lived and your hair will soon return to normal.

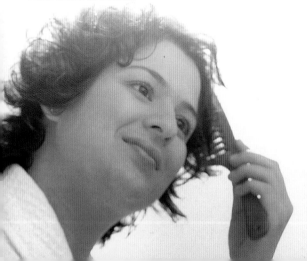

As your pregnancy progresses, and certainly once your baby is born, you probably won't want to bother with a complicated hairstyle, so go for an easily managed style. This will keep your hair looking and feeling healthy throughout your pregnancy and beyond.

Throughout your pregnancy, choose more natural or organic shampoos and conditioners as most commercial products contain a great deal of chemicals. A wet and warm scalp more readily absorbs anything applied to it. You may want to take special care with anti-dandruff shampoos, which contain irritating chemicals. Try some head massage and a conditioning oil treatment instead. Avoid anti-lice shampoos; these contain very strong chemicals, which can pass into the blood stream.

Hair treatments
Although some health professionals are cautious about dyeing or highlighting hair during pregnancy, there's no evidence that these pose any risk to your baby. However, they all contain strong chemicals so if you're at all concerned, avoid colouring hair during the first

trimester and, after that, use only vegetable-based products such as pure henna. Be aware, however, that pregnancy hormones may make your hair react differently to dyes, so you could end up with a colour you weren't expecting.

There's also no evidence to suggest that the chemicals in perms are harmful to you or your developing baby. However, your hair may react unpredictably to them and you could end up with frizzy rather than wavy hair.

Hair relaxers contain strong chemicals so their use is best avoided in pregnancy.

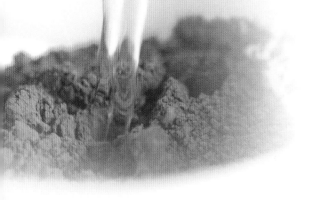

Greasy or dry?

✓ If greasiness is a problem, use special shampoos. Wash hair frequently with a specially formulated shampoo and try not to brush your hair too vigorously, as this will encourage the sebaceous glands in the scalp to produce even more oil.

✓ If your hair becomes dry and flyaway, invest in a hot-oil treatment or deep conditioner to use once a week. Mousse can add volume, improve 'bad-hair days' and keep your style in place. Again, don't brush your hair too much as this will encourage the hair to split.

Tooth and gum care

It's even more important than usual to maintain good dental hygiene throughout pregnancy. If you don't do so already, brush your teeth at least twice a day, ideally after every meal. Throw out your toothbrush as soon as it shows signs of wear. Floss daily but do so gently,

Your eating patterns will affect your teeth, so, if you are now eating several small meals a day (and maybe a snack at night), you will need to clean your teeth more often. Bacteria in your mouth ferment the starches and sugars found in food into acid, which in turn, attacks your teeth. Cleaning your teeth regularly, especially after eating, reduces this bacterial activity.

Bear in mind also that at night, the amount of saliva in your mouth decreases, so midnight snacks should be sugar- and starch-free unless you are prepared to clean your teeth afterwards.

You'll need to see your dentist more regularly than normal during pregnancy – once every six months is advisable. Tell your dentist that you're pregnant, as he or she will want to avoid using X-rays at this time and may advise that any extensive treatment should wait until after your baby is born.

Bleeding gums
The pregnancy hormones circulating in your body will probably cause your gums to swell slightly, making them more susceptible to bleeding during brushing and flossing. They also will make the gums more susceptible to plaque and bacteria. If bleeding gums hurt, you can numb pain with an ice cube or use a little of the homeopathic tincture hypercal.

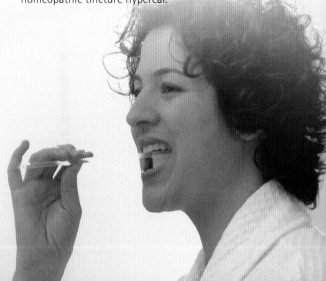

Keeping your mouth in good shape

✓ Clean your teeth regularly, particularly after eating sugary snacks. Take a toothbrush to work with you.

✓ Use a soft-bristled brush, which is less likely to cause your gums to bleed.

✓ Massage your gums gently, making small circular rotations all around with your fingertips, after brushing to encourage blood circulation.

✓ Chew a stick of sugar-free chewing gum when you can't brush after eating as this will help to prevent plaque build-up.

✓ Nibble some reduced-fat Cheddar or Edam cheese as these are good for stimulating saliva that can neutralize mouth acids.

✓ Opt for low-sugar snacks such as vegetable crudités, dips and salsa or raisins, which contain bacteria-suppressing chemicals.

✓ Eat plenty of vitamin C-rich berries and citrus fruit, broccoli and potatoes to strengthen capillary walls and connective tissue, to reduce the risk of bleeding.

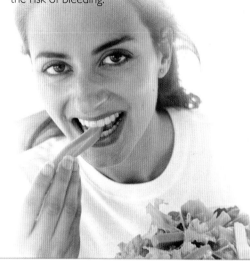

Pregnancy is not the time to

✕ Use lightening fluids, which contain bleach to even out skin colour; use a good quality concealer.

✕ Use anti-wrinkle creams containing vitamin A, as it's possible that the nutrient can be absorbed through the skin and enter the bloodstream. There is strong evidence to suggest that vitamin supplements or medications containing vitamin A can cause birth defects. If you're at all in doubt about what's safe to use, discuss it first with your healthcare provider.

✕ Use hair relaxers as these contain strong chemicals. Although there is no evidence that they are dangerous during pregnancy, there is no proof that they are completely safe, so their use is best avoided.

✕ Undertake semi-surgical procedures including chemical peels and botox and collagen injections because they use concentrated chemicals whose effects on the unborn baby are not known.

✕ Have your teeth whitened. Although no major studies have been done on the effects of using whitening systems – many of which use peroxide or ultraviolet light – until more is known, it's recommended that teeth whitening should be avoided during pregnancy.

✕ Get a tattoo or piercing because of the high risk of infection even if you attend a reputable parlour.

✕ Get breast implants for the first time.

Your changing body shape

During the months of pregnancy, your changing body shape is beautiful evidence of the life growing within you. Alterations that were subtle in the early stages are by now an obvious testament to your unborn child: a thickened waistline, stretched abdomen and breasts heavy in readiness for feeding. But these exciting signs that your body is preparing itself for motherhood can also be difficult to get used to.

If you find you are enjoying the growth of your baby while being uncomfortable with your unfamiliar shape, don't despair. It's perfectly alright to have these feelings: almost every expectant mother does. In fact, negative thoughts are often due to social conditioning – pregnancy means fat means ugly. Yet in many cultures, pregnant women are revered and their bodies thought of as beautiful. Accept that negative thoughts may arise, but understand that you can let these thoughts go while maintaining positive beliefs and visions about your changing shape. Affirmations and visualisations will help you do this: both are powerful tools that can help you turn negative into positive.

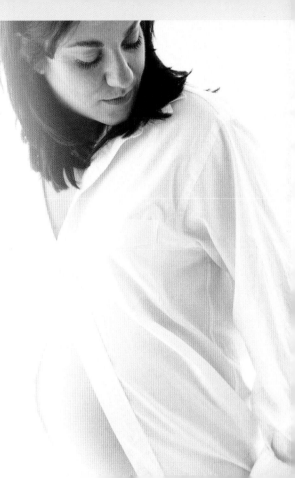

Love your changing body

Use this meditation when you want to

- Overcome the feeling that your body is no longer your own

- Banish fears that you're putting on too much weight (or that you won't be able to lose it once the baby is born)

- Rediscover confidence in your attractiveness and sexuality

How to practise this meditation

At this stage, it may be easier to lie down while you meditate. Choose somewhere quiet and comfortable and, if you are lying on your side, make sure you have a pillow or cushion between your legs to give you proper support. If it's a nice day, lie near an open window so any bird song can be incorporated into your visualisation (see below). Alternatively, lie in a warm bath, with your head supported by a rolled towel and the room lit only by a candle.

The following affirmations, when repeated over and over, will help you see your changing body in a very positive light.

My body is beautiful. It is a growing sign of life within me and is the giver of life.

I am proud of my body. It is beautiful to the eye and sensual to the touch.

I accept what comes up in my thoughts and feelings and am learning to love myself for all of me and for the way I am.

Your transforming body is in itself a very visual image. If you see yourself as beautiful and are proud of your body, others will share in your positive self-image, but if you think of yourself as ungainly and unattractive, then that's what you will be.

To strengthen the efficacy of an affirmation, create an image along the lines of one of the following, personalising it to suit your own needs, if you like. The clearer the image, the better the results. Repeating the affirmation as often as necessary will ensure that the image truly becomes a part of you.

Imagine yourself running easily and freely along a beautiful seashore. You are moving gracefully, in light clothing. You feel the wind in your hair and the sand beneath your feet; you feel as light as a feather and you can turn and twist as much as you wish.

Imagine being relaxed and at ease with yourself. It is a beautiful day and you are walking confidently along a street, proud of your shape, which shows your fertility and enhances your sense of being a woman. You are aware of admiring glances appreciating your body, but have no need to acknowledge them.

COMBATTING 3RD TRIMESTER SIDE EFFECTS

While many women feel great during the last three months, others feel anxious, exhausted and uncomfortable. The weight of your near mature baby can take its toll on your body, resulting in a variety of different complaints from shortness of breath to stress incontinence. There are things you can do to make yourself feel more comfortable; most importantly, you should rest whenever possible and take things easy. Once your baby is born, you will gradually regain your old self.

Fluid retention and swelling

Your body swells due to the accumulation of fluid in the tissues. The swelling is connected to the normal increase in body fluids in pregnancy, and three out of four pregnant women will develop oedema (swelling) at some time. It is common but completely harmless. You are more likely to suffer from it if you are expecting more than one baby, are overweight or if there is a family history of the condition.

Usually the swelling appears in feet and ankles, hands and fingers. To test for oedema on swollen legs, press the skin over your shinbone. A white pitted mark will appear that lasts for over 30 seconds. Oedema is most noticeable at the end of the day or after prolonged standing or sitting and in warm weather.

Swelling could be a sign of pre-eclampsia (see page 239), so you should mention it at your check-ups. A painfully swollen leg that's warm to the touch may be a deep vein thrombosis. Call your healthcare provider immediately if you suspect you have this condition.

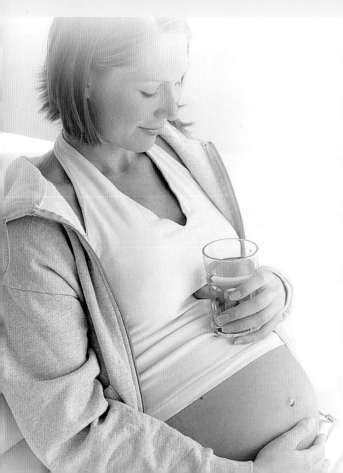

What you can do to help

- Don't stand for long periods. Take regular breaks and sit with your legs elevated.
- Take walks to redistribute the fluid and if you like, yoga postures that will improve the circulation to the legs and feet.
- Lie on your side when resting and keep your legs raised as much as you can. When sitting, don't cross your legs.
- If your hands are swollen, keep your hands elevated above your heart rather than down by your sides.
- Avoid wearing tight clothing, shoes or jewellery.
- Wear support stockings or talk to your healthcare provider about special prescription elastic stockings.
- Drink plenty of water to help to expel excess fluid.
- Don't restrict your salt intake unless your blood pressure is high.

Nasal stuffiness and nosebleeds

High levels of progesterone and oestrogen result in increased blood flow throughout your body, causing the lining of your nasal passages to become swollen. This can lead to congestion and overproduction of mucus. This increased blood flow also puts pressure on your nose's delicate veins, making you more prone to nosebleeds. Nasal stuffiness is likely to get worse before it gets better, after the birth.

What you can do to help
- Increase your intake of fluids.
- Humidify your home, especially your bedroom, at night.
- Prop your head up when you sleep.
- If you have severe congestion, consider breathing steam from a bowl of hot water, or use a saline nasal spray. Don't use medication or medicated nasal sprays unless they are prescribed by your healthcare provider.
- Blow your nose gently to avoid inducing bleeding.
- Eat vitamin C-rich foods, as these will help to strengthen your capillaries.

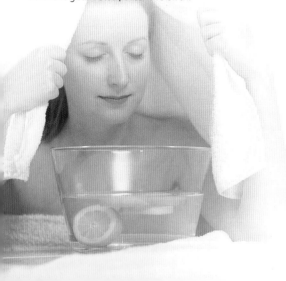

Shortness of breath

Two-thirds of all pregnant women occasionally experience breathlessness. This is a result of a number of things. First of all, it takes an increased effort to simply move around. You also have to absorb about 20 per cent more oxygen and expel more carbon dioxide with each breath as you breathe for your baby. Your enlarged uterus will press against your diaphragm and lungs. And finally the production of progesterone is increased, which speeds up your breathing rate. However, as your baby descends into your pelvis in the final weeks your breathing should improve.

Some medical problems can cause breathlessness such as anaemia, asthma, a chest infection or a heart or lung problem.

What you can do to help

- Relax and try to avoid stress. Try not to panic if you get breathless – it can make it worse.
- Stand tall and allow plenty of room for your chest to expand. Don't slump.
- Avoid lying on your back or sitting or standing for a long time, which can reduce the return of blood to the heart.
- Tightening and releasing your calf and leg muscles or your buttocks about 10-15 times will improve your blood circulation.
- If you experience wheezing, chest pain or blueness of your lips or fingers, get it checked out by your doctor as soon as possible.

Varicose veins

Swollen veins often appear just under the surface of the skin of your legs and sometimes in the vulva and as haemorrhoids around the anus (see page 219). They occur when the uterus puts pressure on the pelvic veins, increasing pressure on the veins in the legs and causing backflow. Blood pools in the veins in the legs causing them to distend.

You may be more likely to get varicose veins if they run in the family, if you're overweight or stand or sit for long periods of time. They're usually painless, but occasionally they may be associated with discomfort, aches or pain. Varicose veins usually regress after delivery, but sometimes not completely. Occasionally, thrombophlebitis (inflammation of a vein due to a blood clot) may develop at the site of a varicosity.

What you can do to help
- Avoid standing still for long periods of time.
- Try to take several rest periods throughout the day so that you can get off your feet.
- Sit with your legs elevated as much as you can.
- If you have to sit still for long periods, move your legs around from time to time to stimulate circulation. Flex your feet up and down to keep the blood from pooling.
- Wear support stockings or talk to your healthcare provider about special prescription elastic stockings but don't wear stockings or socks with tight elastic tops that grip around one part of your leg.
- Try to take a brisk 30-minute walk or swim daily.
- Eat plenty of foods high in vitamin C such as citrus fruits, peppers, strawberries, tomatoes, watercress and potatoes.

Haemorrhoids

Essentially varicose veins of the anal canal, haemorrhoids are caused by the uterus pressing on major blood vessels, making the veins enlarge and swell. Progesterone relaxes the veins, allowing the swelling to increase. Even if you manage to avoid getting haemorrhoids during pregnancy, it is possible to develop them during delivery.

Haemorrhoids sometimes bleed. While this bleeding isn't harmful, if it becomes frequent, talk to your doctor, who may refer you to a colorectal specialist. If your haemorrhoids become very painful, you may want to discuss further treatment.

What you can do to help

- Avoid becoming constipated (see page 168). Straining during bowel movements puts added pressure on the blood vessels.
- Exercise every day to help you to stay regular.
- Sit in a warm bath two or three times a day to help to relieve the muscle spasms that often cause the pain.
- Soothe the area with witch hazel or special pads.
- Speak to your doctor about medications.
- Take pressure off the area by sleeping on your side, and avoid standing for long hours.
- Do pelvic floor exercises (see pages 158 and 191) regularly, as these will help to improve circulation to the area.

Stress incontinence

During the last months of pregnancy, some women begin to leak a little urine when they cough, sneeze, laugh or move suddenly. Referred to as stress incontinence, this is perfectly normal and is caused by the growing uterus putting pressure on the bladder.

Loss of urine also can be a sign of a urinary tract infection and a continuous loss of fluid may be a sign of ruptured membranes (see page 266). If you are not sure about the fluid, give it a sniff. If it doesn't smell like urine or if you suspect a urinary infection or ruptured membranes, get in touch with your healthcare provider.

Stress incontinence may persist after a vaginal delivery so its important to keep the pelvic floor strengthened. Begin exercising again as soon as possible after birth.

What you can do to help

- Practice your pelvic-floor exercises (see pages 158 and 191) regularly to help to strengthen pelvic-floor muscles and support the urinary sphincter.
- Rocking backwards and forwards on the toilet helps to reduce pressure on the bladder so that it can be completely emptied,
- Avoid beverages and foods that can irritate your bladder; these include coffee, citrus juices and fruits, carbonated drinks, alcohol, tomatoes and spicy dishes.
- Keep drinking water otherwise you may suffer from a urinary tract infection or dehydration.
- Go to the toilet more frequently.

Carpal tunnel syndrome

The carpal tunnel in front of the wrist houses the tendons and nerves that run to the fingers. If the hand and fingers swell in pregnancy, the carpal tunnel swells, too, putting pressure on a nerve, which results in pain in the wrist, pins and needles spreading down into all the fingers except the little finger and stiffness of fingers and joints of the hand. These symptoms tend to be worse at night; they usually ease during the day as the joints are used and become more supple.

What you can do to help
- Avoid prolonged typing or using a mouse without wrist support;
- Sleep with your hands raised on a pillow to prevent fluid from building up;
- On waking, drop your hands over the side of the bed and givie them a vigorous shake to disperse fluid and ease any stiffness;
- Wear splints on the wrists.

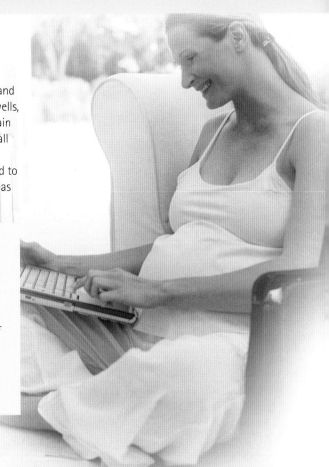

Overcoming sleep problems

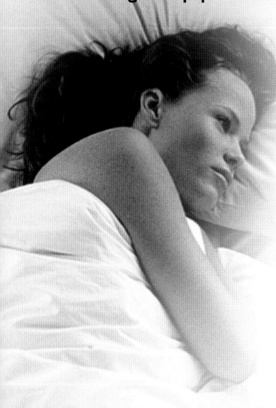

Many women complain of difficulty sleeping during the last few months of pregnancy. This may be due in part to normal anxiety about having a baby, but also may be due to the physical discomforts that can occur later in pregnancy. As your uterus grows, finding a comfortable sleeping position can sometimes be quite a challenge. Sleeping on your back may be uncomfortable as the baby is lying against your spine, which can cause tingling, dizziness and breathlessness, while lying on your side means the baby can use you as a 'springboard', pushing against the mattress.

Your baby now has plenty of movement and will be enjoying moving his arms and legs around. His body clock will not necessarily match with yours, which can mean restless nights. He will now be taking up more room in your uterus, which in turn will press on your bladder, meaning you may want to use the toilet every couple of hours. These frequent trips to the bathroom and commonly occurring night sweats also can disturb deep sleep. Don't be tempted to drink less water during the day to avoid having to get up in the night, because you still need plenty of fluids.

For a more peaceful night, try one or more of the following tips

✓ Keep late-night drinks to a minimum; choose warm milk, which can make you sleepy, or decaffeinated tea or coffee. Cut out late evening drinks if you often get up during the night.

✓ Eat a light evening meal to prevent indigestion and heartburn. Consume carbohydrate-rich foods, such as bread, pasta, rice and potatoes, with your evening meal or have breakfast cereal for supper to help induce sleep.

✓ Have a relaxing bath before bed. Add a couple of drops of an essential oil to the water, such as camomile, which relieves stress and tension.

✓ Ensure your bedroom is conducive to sleep (dark and not too warm), the phone is switched off and your bed is giving you proper support.

✓ Invest in a number of pillows to tuck under your bump, and under and between your legs, making it easier to find a comfortable position.

✓ Avoid reading about labour just before switching off the lights – stick to a book that won't get your thoughts churning!

✓ Keep daytime naps to the morning or early afternoon so that they don't interrupt your nocturnal sleep patterns.

✓ Get plenty of fresh air.

✓ Try to exercise on a regular basis.

Get a good night's sleep

Use this meditation when you want to

- Wind down after a tiring day

- Get to sleep, despite physical discomfort

- Put an end to wakeful hours of worrying

How to practise this meditation

Concentrating on your breathing is one of the best ways to get to sleep. The deeply relaxed state that this type of meditation brings can help slow down your mind and body if you are having difficulty dropping off, and focus your mind on getting back to sleep if you have woken. Before you begin, support your back or legs (if lying on your side) with a cushion or pillow to make you more comfortable. Now, close your eyes and, starting from the top of your head, visually work your way down your body, imagining any tension easing away. Focus on your breathing, counting each breath as you exhale, up to ten, then repeat. Alternatively, silently say 'Sleep' each time you breathe out. Don't worry about how quickly or slowly you are breathing.

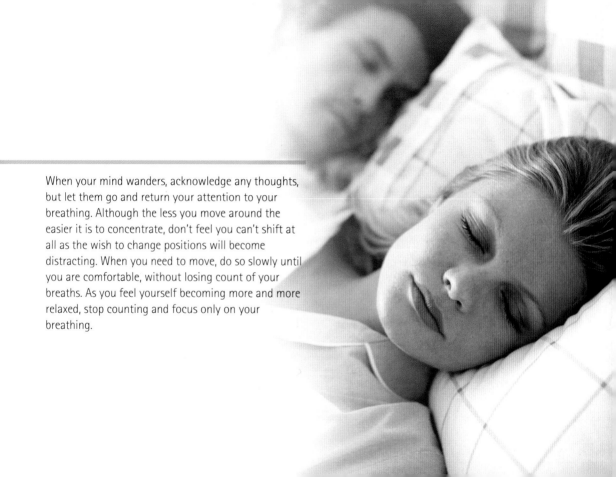

When your mind wanders, acknowledge any thoughts, but let them go and return your attention to your breathing. Although the less you move around the easier it is to concentrate, don't feel you can't shift at all as the wish to change positions will become distracting. When you need to move, do so slowly until you are comfortable, without losing count of your breaths. As you feel yourself becoming more and more relaxed, stop counting and focus only on your breathing.

RELAXATION

For your wellbeing and the health of your baby, you need to take things easy on a regular basis and rest whenever your body demands it – whenever you feel tearful, tired, nauseous or ravenously hungry – in order to maintain your energy supplies. If you are working, you should stop completely by 32 weeks. Women who have to work past 32 weeks are more likely to go into labour prematurely. This advice is particularly pertinent for mothers in their late 30s and 40s.

During the third trimester, many women find they need a siesta after lunch and again on getting home from work. Lie down whenever the urge takes you without feeling guilty as you are only doing what's best for your baby.

At your desk take regular breaks to stretch your limbs: this can stave off back and neck pain, swollen ankles and carpal tunnel syndrome (see page 00). When commuting, try to travel outside the rush hour and always demand a seat. Don't schedule every moment of your journey to be productive. Switch off and daydream: watch people passing, the changing cityscape, trees in bud or leaf and imagine your life in the very same season next year – with a baby.

Helpful relaxing positions

Certain positions not only help you de-stress at home and work but they may help ease your baby into the best position for labour. In the last six weeks before the birth, try to adopt the following forward-leaning relaxation poses for 20 minutes twice a day or more. Elevate your feet when sitting to lessen the chance of developing varicose veins and swollen ankles. To make sure your lower back doesn't arch, place another cushion here to provide support.

Watching tv

Sit on your heels, knees wide open and place pillows beneath your knees and feet and under your buttocks. Pile up large cushions, or a beanbag or birth ball, in front of you, then recline forward onto them, adjusting the support until you feel at ease.

Reading

Get into an all-fours position, hands beneath shoulders, knees beneath hips. Spread your fingers and flatten your palms to the floor, distributing your weight evenly between hands and knees and from right to left. Look down and place the book or magazine slightly forward to elongate your spine (don't let your lower back drop). Every few pages, rock your body forward and back, and circle your weight in one direction, then the other.. When the weight gets too much for your wrists, sink back onto your hips, keeping your knees wide, and rest for a few minutes, arms stretching forward. This relieves back pain.

At a desk

Sit on a cushion to raise your hips higher than your knees. If your chair is uncomfortable or makes your back ache, swap it for a regular dining chair and 'customise' it until you find a position in which you are comfortable. Turn it around, cushion the back and top, and lean forward onto it.

Alternative ways to relax

If you are prone to anxiety, you may like to explore an alternative remedy to help you beat stress. Meditation is a key one, and you will find the ones in this book a great help. Many natural therapies aim to improve the wellbeing of the whole body, not just treat a specific symptom, although each works in a slightly different way. Try one or several of the following, but do consult the advice of a qualified practitioner first as evensome 'natural' remedies are unsafe to use in pregnancy.

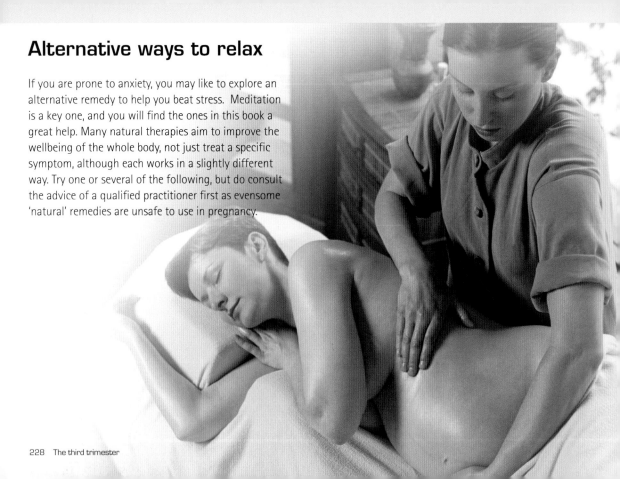

Homeopathy

This therapy treats the whole person – mentally, physically and emotionally – rather than just the symptoms. It works by helping the body to heal itself on the basis of treating like with like. Small amounts of the treatment, that would in larger doses cause the complaint, actually ease it. Remedies are given in different potencies, usually in pilules.

Herbal remedies

The healing properties of plants, trees, flowers and herbs can be accessed in the form of teas, infusions, decoctions or added to a bath. Try a lavender-scented pillow or mustard footbath when you need relaxing.

Flower remedies

These are said to contain the 'energy' imprint of a plant, which works on the vibrations of our own energy patterns, restoring the flow disrupted, for instance, by anxiety. The essences are dropped onto the tongue or taken in water.

Aromatherapy

This technique uses the aromatic oil essences of plants and flowers, diluted in a carrier oil, to heal mentally and physically. Oils can be inhaled via a vaporiser or bath, or absorbed through the skin during massage.

Reflexology

This therapy is based on the principle that each part of the foot corresponds to an area of the body and that massaging certain points on the foot can relieve physical problems.

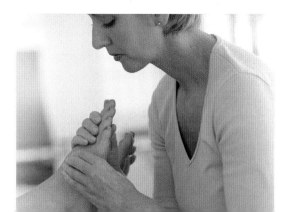

Breathing techniques

Deep, controlled breathing is the essence of relaxation: it can reduce a raised heart rate and regulate blood pressure, help you let go of muscular tension and calm the mind by blocking stressful thoughts. More to the point, it can get you through labour drug-free. The lungs stretch from above the collarbone right down to your diaphragm. Many people use only part of the lungs' capacity for breathing, thus denying their bodies the oxygen they need to perform at their peak, and reducing their resources for coping with stress.

Checking your breathing
Take a few moments to find out whether you have a healthy breathing pattern. Sit down and put your hands on your bump. When you breathe in, you should feel your abdomen expanding to draw air into your lungs and when you breathe out, your abdomen should flatten again. Many people have an inverted breathing pattern and suck their abdomens in when inhaling.

Relaxed shoulders mean relaxed breathing. Try tensing your shoulders by pulling them up towards your ears. Notice how tight your breathing becomes; pulling your shoulders too far downwards or backwards has the same effect. When your shoulders are loose, your breathing is easy. Get in the habit of checking your shoulders regularly throughout the day, especially when you're feeling tense. Let your arms hang down and roll your shoulders backwards and forwards slowly, making sure that they're relaxed so that you can breathe well.

On-the-spot relaxation
Breathe in deeply. When your lungs are full, sigh out gently through your mouth and let the out-breath carry the tension away from the top of your body right down to your toes. When your lungs are ready, let them fill again. Then sigh out gently, relaxing your forehead, jaws, shoulders, hands, stomach and legs. The out-breath is the breath that cleanses your body of stress. If you feel tense at any time remember: sigh out slowly.

Counting the breath

Draw your mind away from troubling thoughts or outside disturbances by following your breath. Counting the breath guides you to follow the action and stops stressful thoughts intruding.

1 Sit comfortably upright. Rest your hands on your thighs (relaxing your shoulders). Close your eyes and start to follow your regular breathing pattern.
2 When you feel at ease, breathe in to a count of four. Pause briefly, then breathe out to a count of four. Take a regular "recovery" breath, if necessary, then repeat the cycle for up to three minutes.
3 When you feel comfortable with the technique and no longer need to take recovery breaths, work on extending the out-breath: breathe in, as before, to the count of four, pause for four, then breathe out to a count of eight.

Progressive Muscle Relaxation

When you feel the need for more relaxation than you can achieve by simply putting up your feet, combine deep breathing with muscle-relaxing exercise. This will give you the greatest benefit in the shortest time. The more you practise muscle relaxation the greater the benefit, as it has a cumulative effect. Ideally, it should be practised twice a day. You'll also find this exercise useful once your baby is born – should you find a few minutes in the day in which to perform it!

The theory behind the exercise is that you learn to appreciate the sensation of relaxation by contrasting it with tension.

Perform the exercise lying on your left side or sit in a chair, feet on the floor. If lying on your left side, bend your top leg forward and rest the knee and thigh on one or two pillows. Fold your upper arm comfortably. Close your eyes.

1 Start at the toes and feet: clench the muscles in the left foot tightly, lifting it a few inches; hold, then release. Feel the weight of your relaxed foot on the floor. Work upward, tightening and releasing your left calf and thigh, then repeat on the right leg. Feel the heaviness of your completely relaxed legs.
2 Tense your buttocks, gripping them and lifting slightly. Hold, then release. Pull your abdominal muscles in to cradle your baby and tense your chest. Let all the muscles in your torso relax, soften and spread.
3 Tense your left arm; clench the hand into a fist, then extend the fingers. Feel the arm shake with tension. Let the arm drop, totally relaxed. Repeat on the right arm. Tense your shoulders, pulling them tightly up and into the neck. Hold, then let everything go as you exhale and release.

4 Screw up your face, pursing your mouth, furrowing your forehead, screwing up your eyes and contracting your ears. Then yawn widely, opening your eyes, ears and mouth as wide as possible. Stick out your tongue. Release, letting go of the gripping in the jaw and forehead. Relax your tongue, ears, nostrils and the back of your scalp.

5 Scan your body from the toes up. When you find an area of tension, imagine it dissolving with the out-breath, and let the region melt into the support of the floor. Picture every part of your body soft and spreading outward and down, becoming heavier and warmer with each exhalation. Relax for up to five minutes. Stretch your limbs before getting up slowly, head last.

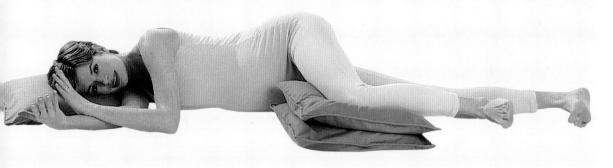

PREGNANCY COMPLICATIONS

Many women suffer minor health problems during pregnancy, but more serious complications occasionally arise, which particularly may affect the third trimester and delivery. When these conditions occur treatment is usually required, so it is important to report any unusual symptoms to your healthcare provider immediately.

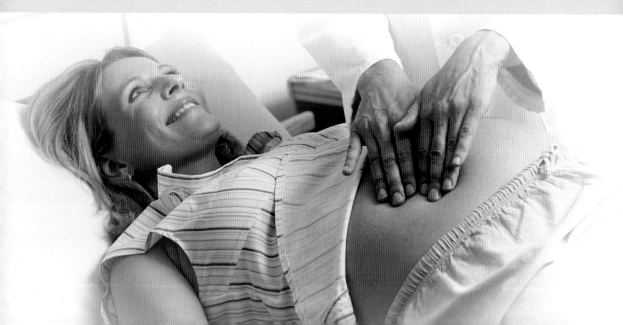

Anaemia

The most common anaemia of pregnancy is dilutional anaemia in which red blood cells do not increase in step with the serum component of blood to sustain a growing baby and thus become diluted.

Iron deficiency is the other major cause. Because you need to produce enough red blood cells for both you and your baby, you need more iron during pregnancy to maintain blood volume. Most women don't have enough stored iron and it's difficult to ingest sufficient amounts. Consequently, a large number of women become anaemic in pregnancy.

Anaemia also can be caused by folic acid deficiency (the B vitamin needed to produce red blood cells), blood loss and chronic illness.

Treatment

During pregnancy, iron deficiency anaemia is treated with an iron supplement. In addition, iron-rich foods — molasses, red meat, kidney beans, spinach, fish, chicken and pork — should form a major part of the diet. Vitamin C increases iron absorption, so iron pills should be taken with orange, tomato or vegetable juice.

In rare cases, a woman may be unable to absorb adequate iron and may require injections of iron preparations. Folic acid or vitamin B12 also may be given. In severe cases, blood transfusions may be needed, especially if labour and delivery are near.

Symptoms
- Fatigue, loss of energy
- Pallor
- Decreased ability to fight illness
- Dizziness, fainting, shortness of breath

Deep vein thrombosis (DVT)

This is a condition which occurs when a blood clot blocks a vein in one of the legs – usually the calf vein or a vein in the upper leg or groin area. Although the greatest risk is generally in the week after birth, particularly if you've had a Caesarean, it is more likely to occur if you engage in extended bed rest before the birth, have varicose veins, are overweight and smoke.

Symptoms
- Pain, tenderness and swelling of the calf, upper leg or groin that does not improve with bed rest
- Swollen area feels warm
- Breathlessness

Treatment
If you suspect you may have DVT, you need to go straight to the hospital, because if left untreated the clot can travel to the lungs causing a pulmonary embolus, which can be life-threatening. A special blood test is available which can confirm the diagnosis and a Doppler ultrasound scan will quickly tell doctors if a DVT is present. Treatment usually consists of blood-thinning injections or medication.

It's easy to confuse DVT with the common and harmless condition of superficial thrombo-phlebitis. Sometimes the small surface veins in the lower legs become red and sore in pregnancy, especially if you're overweight. In this case, only soothing cream and support tights are required.

Gestational diabetes

Unique to pregnancy, in this type of diabetes the body fails to make enough insulin to cope with the increased blood sugar levels. The placenta produces a hormone, human placental lactogen, which acts against insulin and can therefore expose a tendency to diabetes. For women with gestational diabetes, the main complication is that the baby can become very large. Delivery often has to occur no later than 40 weeks gestation.

You're at risk of gestational diabetes if you've had it before, if you're over 35, overweight or Asian, if your previous baby was over 4 kg (8 1b 13 oz), if you have a parent or sibling with diabetes, a previous baby with an abnormality or a previous stillbirth. The diagnosis is based on testing the sugar levels in your blood when fasting and after eating a fixed amount of sugar.

Symptoms
- Sugar in urine
- Excessive thirst
- Excessive urination
- Fatigue

Treatment
Most women with gestational diabetes can control their sugar levels by following a relatively sugar-free diet. For some women this is insufficient, not because they don't stick to the diet but because of the pregnancy itself. These women will need to start having at least twice-daily insulin injections to control their blood sugar. This is managed with the hospital diabetic team, who will teach you how to check your sugar levels and how to give yourself injections.

High blood pressure (hypertension)

If a woman's blood pressure (BP) is raised before pregnancy, this is known as essential hypertension. If a woman's blood pressure is elevated only during pregnancy, this is called pregnancy-induced hypertension (PIH). PIH complicates 10 to 15 per cent of all pregnancies, and is defined as a BP greater than 140/90. It normally develops after 20 weeks, and becomes more common the nearer the delivery date. It is more common in first pregnancies.

Mild high blood pressure may cause no problems. Severe high blood pressure may lead to kidney failure or stroke. The major risk is to the one in four women with PIH who go on to develop pre-eclampsia (see page 239). Many women with pre-eclampsia feel perfectly well and only realize they have this condition because they are told their blood pressure is high.

Symptoms
There are usually no symptoms of high blood pressure until some organs, such as the kidney and eyes, are affected by the decreased blood supply that can accompany hypertension. Because untreated hypertension can eventually lead to serious complications, blood pressure checks are routine at antenatal visits.

Treatment
Lifestyle changes may be prescribed including reducing strenuous activities and cutting down on work.. Relaxation activities including meditation, yoga, aromatherapy massage and reflexology may be recommended. In severe cases, bed rest may be advised

Hypertensive medication may be administered either orally or via an intravenous infusion.

Pre-eclampsia

A syndrome that occurs only in pregnancy, pre-eclampsia is characterised by high blood pressure, protein in the urine and increased swelling of the legs and feet. Pre-eclampsia affects eight to 10 per cent of pregnancies, and 85 per cent of these are first-time pregnancies. Higher risk mothers are those over 40 or teenaged, who are overweight, or who have diabetes, a history of blood-pressure problems or previous pre-eclampsia, or kidney or rheumatology disorders, or who are expecting twins or more.

Symptoms
- Sudden excessive lower leg oedema (swelling) or excessive weight gain
- Persistent headaches
- Blurred vision, flashing lights or spots before your eyes
- Upper abdominal pain on right side of the body, just below ribcage

Treatment
The cause of pre-eclampsia remains unknown, though a protein is suspected, and consequently no treatment has been consistently shown to prevent or treat it. Birth is the only cure, with induced delivery for women who are close to their due dates or who are severely affected. If it is still early in the pregnancy or if pre-eclampsia is mild, blood-pressure tablets can help to reduce blood pressure. Low-dose aspirin – 75 mg daily – and possibly calcium, may reduce your risk of developing it. Attend all your check-ups, so any problems can be detected early. Try not to get stressed, as this can raise blood pressure. Cut down on sodium and fat; eat more calcium-rich foods, fruit and vegetables, and drink plenty of water. You may be asked to monitor your blood pressure so you can spot any dramatic change.

Eclampsia

Pre-eclampsia can develop into eclampsia, a rare but very serious condition involving convulsions, seizures and possible coma, which can occur before, during or post labour. Due to modern obstetric care, this is very unlikely to arise but if it does so, the baby will be delivered no matter its gestational age.

Symptoms
- Seizures
- Convulsions
- Possible coma

Treatment
Eclampsia is a medical emergency, and oxygen and drugs will be given to the mother to prevent any further seizures occurring. Urgent delivery of the baby, generally by Caesarean section, is usually required to enable proper treatment of the mother.

HELLP syndrome

A life-threatening condition, HELLP syndrome is a unique variant of pre-eclampsia. It stands for its characteristics: H is for haemolysis (the breaking down of red blood cells); EL for elevated liver enzymes; and LP for low platelet count. HELLP syndrome occurs in tandem with pre-eclampsia, but because some of its symptoms can occur before those of pre-eclampsia they can be mistaken for other conditions. In the United Kingdom, eight to 10 per cent of all pregnant women develop pre-eclampsia. Between two and 12 per cent of these go on to suffer from HELLP syndrome. Older white women with more than one child are most at risk of getting HELLP.

Symptoms

Headache, nausea, vomiting, and abdominal soreness and pain in the right upper section – from liver distention. Other symptoms that may be present include: visual disturbances, bleeding, swelling, hypertension and protein in the urine.

Treatment

The only effective treatment for women with HELLP syndrome is delivery. The quicker pre-eclampsia is detected and managed, the better the outcome for mother and baby.

Symphysis pubis dysfunction (SPD)

In pregnancy, the hormone relaxin loosens all the pelvic ligaments supporting the pelvic girdle joints (one of which is the symphysis pubis) to allow the baby easier passage at birth. However, these ligaments can loosen too much, making the pelvis move and sometimes allowing the bones to separate, due to the weight of the baby.

SPD can develop at any time from the first trimester onward particularly if you've been immobile for a long time or if you are overactive. It also may occur after an activity such as swimming breaststroke or lifting something incorrectly.

Symptoms
- Pain, usually in the pubis and/or the lower back, but can be in groin, inner thighs, hips and buttocks
- Pain is made worse when weight is on one leg
- A sensation of the pelvis separating
- Difficulty when walking

Treatment
Unfortunately, SPD is untreatable during pregnancy as it's due to the effect of hormones. The condition should improve, however, as your body returns to its pre-pregnancy state. In the meantime great care should be taken not to make SPD worse.

Avoid putting weight on one leg as much as possible – sit down to get dressed, get into the car by putting your buttocks on the seat first, and then lifting your legs into the car. Avoid breast stroke when swimming and keep your knees together when turning over in bed. If the pain is severe, ask your healthcare provider about painkillers and arrange to see a physiotherapist, who may advise a pelvic support belt.

Special care needs to be taken during labour and birth. Good birth positions are on all fours, kneeling up against the back of the bed, or side-lying with the top leg supported.

Antenatal classes

If you haven't done so already, book your antenatal classes. They are much more than just a 'coffee morning with the girls'. They should cover what happens during labour and birth, when to call your healthcare provider, relaxation and breathing techniques, pain relief choices, Caesareans, tips on breastfeeding and care of your newborn. They also offer the opportunity to talk about your pregnancy and baby as much as you want without fear of sending others to sleep!

Encourage your partner to accompany you, too. This will help him understand what you will be going through, encourage you to practise your breathing and other exercises at home and teach him how to support you during labour.

Childbirth classes usually begin at around 28 to 32 weeks. Depending on what you feel you need, you can attend classes spanning a number of weeks, or brush up your knowledge at a one-off refresher session. Classes are often held in the evenings and at weekends and are usually conducted by a midwife.

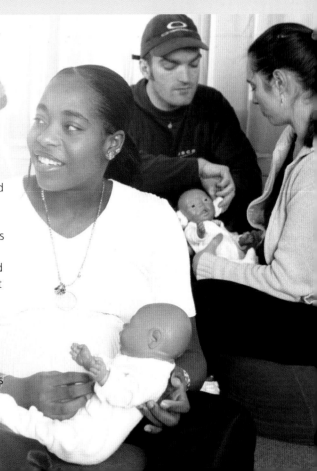

Choosing a class

Ask doctors, midwives, friends or family for recommendations, and find out what classes are available in your area. Health service classes are usually offered by hospitals, healthcare centres and doctors' surgeries. They are run by midwives or health visitors, sometimes with input from a doctor if there is something medical on the agenda. They are free, but are often conducted in large groups, possibly making it harder to make friends with other prospective parents.

Private childbirth classes are usually held in someone's home, or a community setting of some sort, and are run by a teacher trained by the organization offering the classes, who may or may not be a health professional. Some will allow you to sit in on a session so that you can decide if it's right for you. An ideal class size is around five to seven couples – this is large enough to ensure good discussion but small enough so that everyone can benefit from individual attention during sessions.

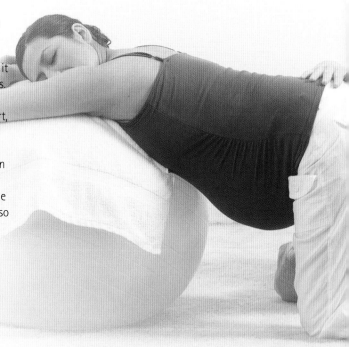

Finding the right teacher

Many private childbirth teachers approach the subject from a specific angle or philosophy, so it's important to find a teacher who shares your views on childbirth. At the same time, approaching different classes with an open mind will help you to learn about different approaches to labour and birth so that you can make informed choices, which really suit you.

National Childbirth Trust (NCT)

The classes are taught by NCT-trained antenatal teachers and take place in the last three months of pregnancy. The classes are for small groups of couples and offer practical information and a chance to talk through your feelings.

Active Birth

Specialising in yoga and relaxation for pregnancy and water births, these classes focus on preparing you for birth in a modern birthing environment.

Lamaze International Inc

Childbirth teachers with Lamaze certification encourage active birth and specific breathing patterns to distract from the pain of labour.

Bradley Certification

These classes focus on husband-coached, 'natural' childbirth with emphasis on diet, antenatal exercise, and inner focus to cope with the pain of labour.

Most private classes are run over six to eight sessions, in the last few weeks of pregnancy. In some areas you may find 'labour and birth' weekends or days, where you attend for one or two long sessions.

Well Mother

Therapists teach shiatsu, massage, postures, and ante- and post natal exercise to both partners to improve the birth experience and to enable parents to bond early with their developing child.

Looking ahead to motherhood

It's natural to have some worries about how your life is going to change and how you will adapt, but being aware that your life will change is the first step to an exciting new life. No one can give you any guarantees, but the fact that most women have more than one child is a good indicator that labour and motherhood is obviously worthwhile! What mothers, midwives and doctors all agree on is that the more prepared you are, the more easily you will cope.

It's important to feel relaxed and calm during the last few weeks. It is now that you need to focus on yourself and your own needs. If you haven't stopped work already, you should soon be on maternity leave, which will leave you more time to yourself. If you are planning to go back to work full or part time, you'll need to arrange some form of childcare, and returning to work will be a lot easier if you feel happy and confident about this.

Meditation can help you to relax, focus on your needs and calm any worries you may have. If you feel peaceful and at ease, then so will your baby who can benefit from your relaxed pace and tranquil thoughts.

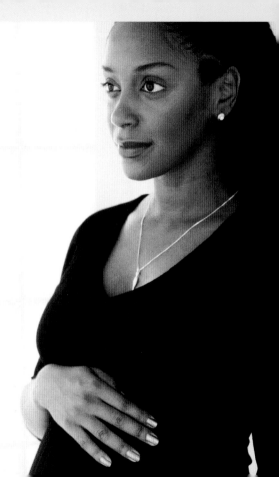

Childcare options

Ask your health visitor, family and friends for recommendations, and get a list of registered childminders from your local authority. Bear in mind that the most important factor is to ensure the safety and well-being of your baby. Licensing, training certificates, references and any facility that you are considering should always be double-checked.

Take time to research your options. Your baby needs to be with someone that you and your partner both like and trust, otherwise the arrangement will fall apart. Your basic choices are:

Parent at home

Obviously this is the ideal option. One of you stays at home to look after the baby, or you both work different hours so that the care can be shared.

Family

Having your mother or another relative looking after your baby can be an excellent childcare solution, providing your baby with continuity of care.

Nanny

In-home care can be expensive, but if you have more than one child it becomes more economical. There's no doubt that one-on-one care during the first year of life is very beneficial, but that depends on having a reliable, experienced nanny who's in tune with a child's physical and emotional needs.

Nurseries

These work well for children of any age, as long as they're of a high standard. However, not all nurseries take babies under the age of 12 months.

Childminder

This is offered by people who are licensed to offer childcare in their homes, possibly in combination with looking after their own children. This arrangement will provide playmates and a family environment for your child, and has the advantage of her having the same caregiver and being in a small group.

Become focused

Use this meditation when you want to

- Prepare yourself for the long-term (motherhood) and not just for the immediate future (labour)

- Examine your expectations about what lies ahead

- Reassure yourself you will retain your self-identity

How to practise this meditation

This technique will help to focus your thoughts so that when the future becomes reality, you will be better prepared to deal with any situation calmly and positively.

Start by picking an object that is beautiful to you – a vase of flowers, the flame of a candle, a tree in the garden – and sit or lie in front of it. As you focus on each out-breath, you will be aware of noises around you – a neighbour talking, a car starting, or somebody's radio – but just acknowledge these are present, don't let them distract you.

Observe the details of what you are looking at: the texture of a petal, the way the flame dances in movement, the rustle of leaves as the tree sways in the

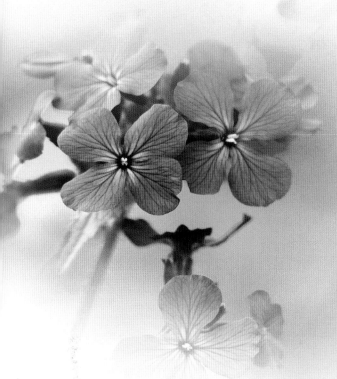

wind. Silently name what you are seeing with each out-breath (for instance, petal). Repeat a few times and then move on to another aspect (e.g. blue) and then another (say, moving), until you feel as if you are becoming part of what you are looking at, part of the beauty. Slowly come out of the meditation and be aware of how your mind has focused and how relaxed your body feels.

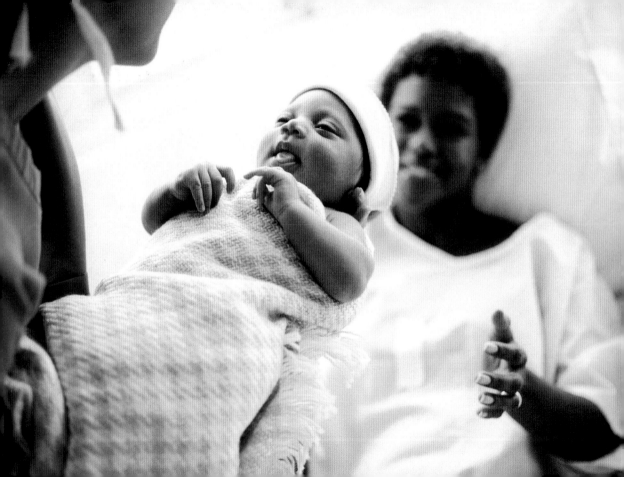

Chapter 5

Labour and delivery

THE FINAL STAGES

These last few weeks are among the most exciting times of your pregnancy, and the days can now appear frustratingly long as you impatiently wait for the new arrival. The excitement also is often tinged with anxiety about labour and how you will cope with life beyond labour – the hard but fulfilling job of looking after a baby. As your due date approaches you'll want to prepare yourself, your partner and your baby for the birth. Now is the time to look at things you can do that will help you to be comfortable, and to address concerns you may have about giving birth.

Although childbirth is not without discomfort, women have managed it throughout history. Learning as much as you can about labour can help you overcome any exaggerated fears you may have about it and thus make the experience a more positive one.

Babies rarely appear on their due dates, so it's a good idea to take note of the signs that labour is beginning – since the majority of babies are born two weeks either side when they are expected.

Preparing yourself

Your pregnancy and labour together comprise a very personal and unique period in your life – yet many women tend to feel anxious as they feel they are not in control. Fears about being unable to cope with the pain, having an epidural (see page 281) or not being allowed to move around can justifiably gain great significance. But, within the confines of safety, you should be able to do what you want during your labour.

Create a birth plan

Help yourself by being prepared. Together with your partner, read up about all the options available to you and decide on a birth plan that you feel happy with. Don't be pressured into making any decisions you're not sure about – be assertive about what you want. Things to include are who you would like to be present at birth, whether you agree to induction and monitoring, how you want labour to be managed, and what sort of pain relief you'd like.

Talk to your midwife or consultant well before your due date and explain what you would like. If you're having your baby in hospital, visit the delivery room,

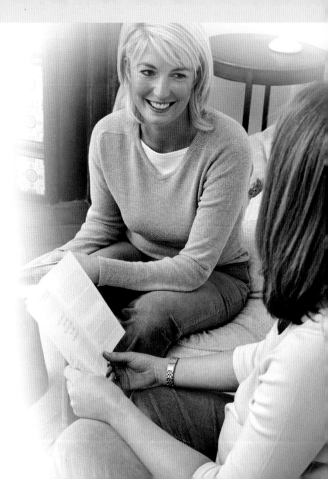

find out about the hospital's policy on giving epidurals and what the rate is for Caesarean sections. And remember that the medical staff at hospital are there to make sure the delivery is as safe and supportive as possible for both you and the baby.

Being in control is not only about knowing what you want, but also acknowledging that this may have to change if things don't go according to plan. No birth is perfect, so the more open-minded you and your partner are about the way the birth might go, the more you will be able to cope if things don't work out the way you wished.

Emotional fears can affect the birth in a very direct physical way. If you aren't prepared for the discomfort of normal contractions, you may believe that something is wrong and become frightened. This can disrupt your breathing, increase the tension – and therefore pain – in your muscles, and may even decrease the flow of oxytocin, the hormone that causes the uterus to contract. Learning about labour and good birth support can help you to work with contractions rather than resist them.

Tips for keeping comfortable

✓ Wear light, loose clothing as you'll be feeling hotter than normal. This is due to increased fat deposits and an increased metabolism.

✓ Try to get as much sleep as possible. Supplement your nightly sleep with naps, especially if you're being woken by trips to the toilet.

✓ Keep your body hydrated by drinking plenty of water so that you cope better with your faster metabolism and to relieve swelling feet and legs.

✓ Take a break whenever you can. If you have swelling in your feet and legs, sit down and put your feet up on a stool for 10 to 15 minutes, three times a day.

✓ Increase your intake of protein as plenty of milk, eggs, meat and fish can alleviate some of the problems with late pregnancy.

Be in control

Use this meditation when you want to

- Feel empowered about the impending birth

- Quell your nerves about what labour will be like

- Remind yourself that your beautiful baby will make all the discomfort and waiting worthwhile

How to practise this meditation

Pick an affirmation that summarises how you would like to feel, such as:

- I am in control
- I want what is best for my baby
- What is good for my baby is good for me
- My mind and body are calm

Then sit or lie down, making yourself as comfortable as possible. Focus on your breathing, becoming aware of how it slows and regulates, and silently repeat your affirmation. If you do this daily, your affirmation will become part of your subconscious and enter your conscious mind when needed.

mini meditation
Become aware of your senses

Use the following for a minute or two anytime you start to feel overwhelmed by fears. Begin by focusing on what's happening around you. For instance, as you lie in the bath, notice the sensation of the water moving against your body, its heat, your toes pressed against the end of the bath. Don't stop whatever you're doing, just be aware that you are doing it. You could concentrate on one sense, silently repeating the word 'Touch' or 'Sound' to draw you away from unproductive worries and calm you down.

Going overdue

Extra days or weeks past your due date may provide crucial extra resting time before the birth. Only 5 per cent of women deliver on their due date, with the majority giving birth a little later. Your baby is expected to be born within two weeks either side of the due date, so a pregnancy is only considered officially overdue after 42 weeks.

A first pregnancy is prolonged, on average, eight days past the due date. The average second baby is born three days late. Poor positioning of the baby's head, i.e. if it is in the occiput posterior position – the head facing away from the mother's tailbone – also can delay the baby's descent.

A small number of pregnancies outlive the placenta's ability to nourish the baby. Since this can cause problems for the baby, your midwife or doctor may suggest special precautions after 40 weeks to ensure that your baby is doing well.

Kick-count sheets

You should expect to count at least ten movements over a period of 12 hours during the day (see page 187). If you do not, or if your baby seems less active than normal, call your midwife or go to the hospital immediately.

Fetal heart rate monitoring

This is usually carried out by your midwife at the clinic or in the hospital delivery suite.

A biophysical profile

This is an ultrasound that measures your baby's limb and lung movement, and the amount of amniotic fluid.

If your pregnancy approaches 42 weeks, your healthcare provider will discuss the use of induction to start labour (see page 289).

Important phone numbers	
Birth partner	
Doula	
Doctor/midwife	
Hospital	
Taxi	
Relatives	
Maternity nurse	
Nappy service	

Preparing your baby for birth

As your abdomen enlarges and the long-awaited birth of your baby is soon to become a reality, the bond between you both is strengthening. While you are mentally and physically preparing yourself, so too is your baby. At about thirty-six weeks, the baby's head usually engages or drops down into the pelvis in readiness for birth (although this may not happen until a bit later), and all five of the infant's senses are perfectly developed in preparation for life in the outside world.

Babies cry when they're unhappy or want something, so it's not surprising most cry in protest at birth. But some women say so strong was the bond formed in the uterus that their baby made no whimper, only gazing intently up at mother.

Even after a straightforward delivery, it will be a shock for your baby to leave the warm, dark, watery environment of your uterus and enter a bright hospital room, full of strange people. And a more difficult birth – involving ventouse, forceps or a Caesarean delivery, for example – will be even more traumatic. Although there is only a limited amount you can do truly to prepare your baby for the arduous voyage through the birth canal, the more calm, relaxed and prepared you both feel, the more easily you will both cope with the actual birth.

Using visualisation

Your mind is a powerful tool that can be used to reach your baby. Visualisation can have a large part to play in helping you connect with your baby. The more you can 'see' your baby, even if just in your mind's eye, the more you will feel that birth is a process involving both your efforts. If you can work with your baby rather than feeling your body is no longer yours to control, you will find labour and delivery more manageable – even pleasurable. If you can imagine your baby moving further down the birth canal with every contraction, then the accompanying discomfort could be eased by the knowledge that your baby is one step closer to being born. You can use the following as a means of communication in the run-up to your due-date, letting positive thoughts of peace and tranquillity flow through your body and envelop your baby. Sit in a

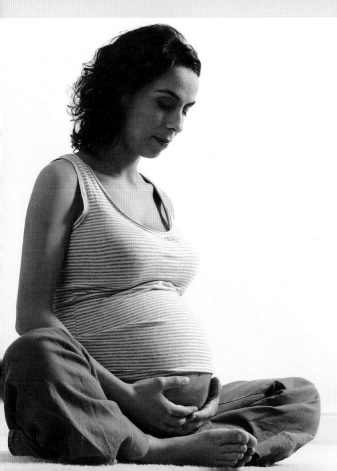

quiet place and breathe gently in and out. Place your hands on your abdomen and focus on your baby – maybe you will feel her kicking or turning. As you breathe, visualise your hands cradling your baby through your abdomen. In your mind or out loud, try to communicate with her, telling her how much you are looking forward to seeing her. Try and explain what her birth journey will be like and how you will work with her to make it as comfortable as possible.

Helping your baby to turn

Visualisation also may be helpful when your baby is lying transverse or breech – less favourable positions for birth. According to Dr. Juliet DeSa Souza, if on an empty stomach you concentrate on relaxing your abdomen while visualising your baby turning head down, there is a good chance she will do so. The visualisation should be practised for 10 minutes twice a day for two to three weeks.

Reassure your baby

Use this meditation when you want to

- Communicate with your baby

- Stimulate your child for the journey that lies ahead

- Ready your baby for life outside the uterus

How to practise this meditation

You can use this not only as a daily meditation, when you are sitting or lying down, but also as a mini meditation, to be incorporated into your day as and when you have a spare minute or so. Begin by focusing on your breathing. As you start to breathe more deeply, imagine each inhalation passing down from your nose to your baby, carrying energising oxygen for the journey ahead. Feel your mind begin to calm down with each out-breath and notice your body begin to relax, the tension ebb out from your joints and muscles and feel your limbs loosen. Now repeat one of the following affirmations out loud.

- Mummy loves you
- All is well
- We two are one

Alternatively, you can repeat a mantra, choosing a
sound that conveys all you want for a positive delivery
for both you and your baby. If you perform this
meditation often enough in your last trimester, your
unborn baby will begin to recognise the words, so you
can use the same affirmation or mantra when you first
hold your baby in your arms – this will be very
comforting to him or her.

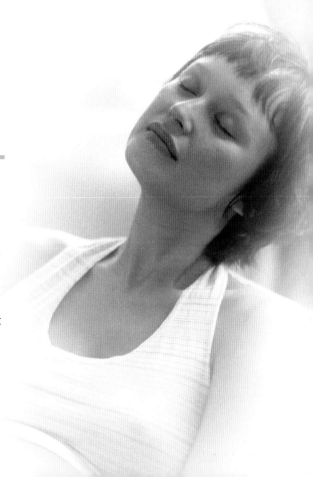

Packing your bags

You should prepare a bag or bags with all the essentials you and your newborn will need in hospital about three weeks before your due date. You also should pack things to take into the delivery room, to help you through labour.

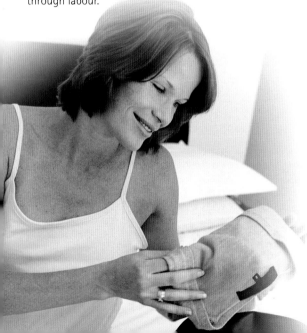

Hospital needs

- ❑ Toothbrush, toothpaste and mouthwash
- ❑ Toiletries
- ❑ Hairbrush, clips and bands
- ❑ Dressing gown, nightgowns and underwear
- ❑ Maternity sanitary pads
- ❑ Breastfeeding supplies: nursing bra, breastfeeding pads, purified lanolin for nipples
- ❑ Watch with a second hand for timing contractions
- ❑ Change for telephone calls, parking and snacks
- ❑ Mobile phone
- ❑ Camera or video equipment
- ❑ Food and drink for your birth partner
- ❑ Slippers and heavy socks for cold feet
- ❑ Changing bag, nappies and baby clothes
- ❑ Birth announcement cards, address list and a pen
- ❑ Baby book for footprints and signatures

Labour aids

❑ A favourite small ornament to focus on
❑ Calming music that you have used before
❑ Comfortable cushions for support
❑ An aromatherapy scented handkerchief
❑ An atomiser water spray to freshen your face
❑ A flannel or sponge to cool you down
❑ Mirror to watch baby emerge
❑ A book or magazine to take your mind off labour if your contractions slow down
❑ Food and snacks to keep you going
❑ Water or juices to keep you hydrated
❑ Extra cushions to prop you up
❑ Lotion or powder for massage
❑ Cold and warm packs for back relief

Going home essentials

❑ Loosely-fitting clothes, including comfortable shoes
❑ Bag for carrying home gifts and hospital supplies
❑ Infant car seat
❑ Going home outfit for your baby: vest, nightgown or all-in-one suit, socks, shawl and a sleep or pram suit, if cold
❑ Nappies and baby wipes

Signs of approaching labour

In the days or weeks before your baby's birth you may have a number of symptoms of your body's preparation for labour. If you are a first-time mum, these physical changes can begin weeks before true labour. With subsequent babies, these changes are more likely to happen closer to the birth.

Engagement

As the lower part of your uterus softens and expands, your baby's head descends lower into your pelvis. This is known as engagement or 'dropping', and when it happens you'll find that you have more space to breathe. Any heartburn symptoms you've had may be eased, and you won't feel uncomfortably full after a meal. Engagement usually occurs between two and four weeks before labour starts if it's your first baby; with subsequent pregnancies it often occurs as labour is about to begin.

Pelvic pressure

Once your baby's head is settled in your pelvis, you may experience some minor discomforts. You'll probably need to pass water and have bowel movements more frequently because of the pressure that your baby is placing on your bladder and bowels. The relaxation of your joints and ligaments may make your pubic bones and back ache, and you may experience sharp twinges as your baby presses down on your pelvic floor. Compression of pelvic blood vessels can cause your legs and feet to swell. Pelvic rocks and lying on your left side can help to relieve some of this pelvic pressure. To perform pelvic rocks, get down on your hands and knees and slowly round your shoulders and back while keeping your head down and your adomen and buttocks tight. Hold this position briefly before straightening the back and raising the head. Repeat 10 times, twice a day or whenever you feel pressure.

Vaginal discharge

Many women experience increased vaginal secretions as the cervix softens. This discharge is usually like egg white, but it can be tinged pink.

A yellow or frothy discharge may signal an infection, so you should report it to your healthcare provider. You also should contact your healthcare provider if you experience a sudden gush of fluid, which could be your waters breaking. If they are stained yellow, green or brown, that means they contain meconium, your baby's bowel movement, and could signal fetal distress.

Nesting instinct

If in the last month you find yourself seized with a sudden desire to empty drawers, clear out closets, and scrub the house from top to bottom, you're simply experiencing what's known as the 'nesting instinct', an inbuilt maternal urge to prepare the home for the imminent arrival of the baby.

While you may want to make the most of this burst of energy, take care not to overdo it. You need to conserve your strength for labour.

Braxton Hicks contractions

Named after the doctor who first identified them, Braxton Hicks aren't true contractions, but 'practice' ones, designed to stretch the lower part of your uterus – enabling your baby's head to settle into your pelvis – and to soften and thin the cervix. In the run-up to labour, these practice contractions can intensify, giving you a tightening or 'balling up' sensation in your abdomen. Lying down usually helps to ease any discomfort.

Shivering or trembling

You may find yourself shivering or trembling for no apparent reason when labour or pre-labour symptoms arrive – often without any sensation of cold or weakness. This can be a result of stress hormones or an alteration in progesterone levels.

Diarrhoea

Prostaglandins, which are the body chemicals released in the process of early labour, may trigger episodes of loose bowel movements.

The onset of labour

The exact cause of the onset of labour remains unknown. The most widely held theory is that your baby produces substances that change pregnancy hormones. Alternatively, you may develop an increasing sensitivity towards the end of pregnancy to substances in the body that produce uterine contractions.

How do you know you're in labour if there's no clearly defined start to it? This is the question that every pregnant woman worries about, but you can rest assured that when the time comes, you will know. Although the only true sign that labour has started is the onset of regular contractions that cause your cervix to dilate, there are other signs that labour is imminent.

Mucus plug and bloodstained show

As the cervix softens, shortens and begins to dilate, the mucus plug that has sealed the cervix for most of your pregnancy is dislodged. This is called a bloodstained show – or sometimes just a 'show' – and usually appears as a small amount of bright red or brownish mucus. A show may also appear as a heavier discharge or it may simply be unnoticeable. Though a show can be a sign that labour's imminent, it can occur as much as six weeks before the birth. However, if you have a show, you should contact your healthcare provider right away for advice.

Rupture of membranes

The amniotic sac containing the fluid around your baby usually ruptures – known as the 'waters breaking' – at some point during labour. Occasionally, however, it may rupture before contractions begin in earnest. Most women go into labour within 24 hours of their waters breaking, as the rupture causes the release of prostaglandins, contraction-stimulating substances. Sometimes a woman may have been having contractions before her waters break but has not been aware of them. Once the waters break, contractions can intensify, as the baby's presenting part (the part that will be born first) now presses directly onto the dilating cervix.

If your waters break at home, make a note of the time it broke and its consistency, and notify your healthcare provider. Amniotic fluid is usually clear and

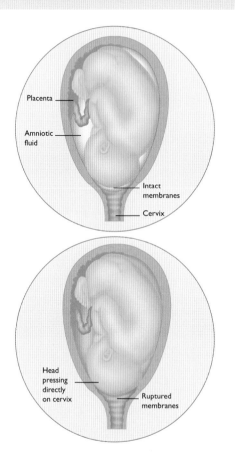

Placenta

Amniotic fluid

Intact membranes

Cervix

Head pressing directly on cervix

Ruptured membranes

odourless, and once the bag of water has ruptured at term, it will go on leaking until delivery. If you're preterm, or if your baby was felt to be un-engaged or high in the pelvis at your last examination, your healthcare provider may recommend that you go into the hospital to be assessed before contractions start. Once your waters break it's important not to put anything into your vagina as there is a possible risk of infection. Showers are preferable to baths until active labour has begun and your baby has been assessed by your healthcare provider.

If you're aware of something pulsing in the vagina after your waters break, this may be a prolapsed cord, so call your healthcare provider immediately and go to the hospital right away.

Regular contractions

Identifiers of true labour are that the cervix steadily dilates (opens out) and there are regular contractions. Early contractions are sometimes called 'false' labour, because they occur only intermittently as they prepare the uterus for true, progressive labour. These early contractions stretch the lower uterus to accommodate the baby as she moves down into it. They also soften the cervix, but do not result in cervical change as regular contractions do. Labour aids or narcotic analgesia may help your body to relax and allow the uterus to work more efficiently.

At some point, any brief, irregular contractions are replaced by ones that have a rhythmic pattern and longer length. These contractions are likely to be progressively contracting the upper uterus while stretching the lower part and opening the cervix. By this mechanism, the powerful upper uterus muscles push the baby through the stretchable lower uterus.

Sometimes back labour occurs. If you experience back pain every 5 minutes, call your healthcare provider and go to the hospital.

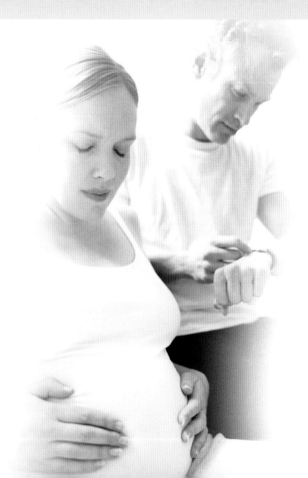

True or false labour?

Contractions are the one sure way to tell if you're in labour or not.
Use this chart to find out if your contractions are the real thing.

True labour	False labour
Contractions have a regular pattern – coming every 5 minutes.	Contractions are irregular – coming every 3 minutes, and then every 5 to 10 minutes.
Contractions become progressively stronger.	Contractions don't intensify with time. Contractions may recede with changes in activity or position.
Contractions don't abate when walking or resting.	
Contractions may be accompanied by a show.	Contractions usually not accompanied by increased mucus or bloodstained show.
Progressive cervical dilatation.	No significant cervical change is detectable.

Going to hospital

The early part of labour can take hours. If you're not in any real discomfort, it's best to stay at home in familiar surroundings where there's plenty to do to distract yourself. If you're in a lot of discomfort, however, you may want to go to the hospital sooner. As a rough guide, aim to go to hospital when contractions are so intense that you're unable to hold a conversation during one and if you've been having regular contractions for over an hour – 5 minutes apart, each lasting 45 to 60 seconds. Intense contractions that are less than 3 minutes apart are often a signal that birth is very near. If you've given birth before, bear in mind, that, on average, second babies arrive in half the time that first babies take.

If your waters break in the midst of regular contractions, this may be a signal to go to hospital. If your waters break before regular 5-minute contractions occur, call your healthcare provider for advice. If you aren't sure whether it's false or real labour, don't feel embarrassed about going to the hospital to be assessed or asking your midwife to check you. It can be easy to misinterpret the signs of labour,

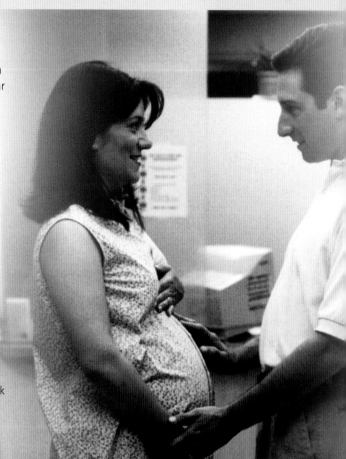

especially with a first pregnancy, and it's better to err on the side of caution.

Arrival procedures

While admissions procedures for hospitals vary greatly, the same things still have to happen once you're admitted. Generally, most women are asked to go to the maternity ward or delivery suite at once, although at a few hospitals you may be asked to go to the casualty department so you can be taken to your room in a wheelchair. Remember to take your pregnancy records with you. You may then be taken to a labour and delivery suite, or the room where you will give birth, where a midwife will assess your progress by carrying out the following procedures.

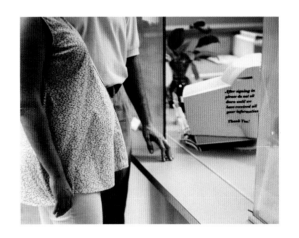

Vital signs

Your pulse, blood pressure, breathing and temperature will be checked repeatedly throughout labour. You'll also be asked about your contractions, whether your waters have broken, and whether you've recently eaten.

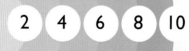

Internal examination

You'll have an internal examination to see whether your cervix is dilated. During labour, the cervix usually dilates at a minimum of 1 cm an hour up to a maximum of 10 cm (see above). If you're in early labour and everything's fine, you may be sent home until you go into active labour.

Brief history

You'll be asked what sort of pregnancy you've had and what sort of pain relief you want to have if you make that decision. You'll probably be given a hospital gown to change into, although some hospitals will allow you to wear your own clothes if you want to.

Monitoring

Your contractions and your baby's heart rate will be monitored in some way – either by an external fetal monitor or a hand-held ultrasound device.

An intravenous line

You may have an intravenous line (IV) inserted if you have had a previous Caesarean or could be at risk of bleeding after the birth. An IV is also needed if you have an epidural later. You may have a blood sample taken for your blood group and an anaemia test.

Fetal monitoring

Devices can be used to check the baby's progress during labour. One of the most common types is the external fetal monitor, consisting of electrodes placed on your abdomen. These are hooked up to a machine that displays or prints out readings of your baby's heartbeat and your contractions.

Some hospitals monitor all women with these monitors continuously in labour. But some studies have shown that it can lead to an increase in unnecessary Caesareans, because the readings were misinterpreted and the monitors indicated that there was a problem where there wasn't. For this reason, if you have had a low-risk pregnancy and birth is assumed also to be low risk, you may be checked with a fetal monitor intermittently, or the baby's progress may be measured with a Doppler (a hand-held ultrasound device).

If your healthcare providers need a more detailed picture of your baby's condition, they may want to monitor your baby internally by passing an electrode through your vagina and attaching it to your baby's scalp to measure the heartbeat. Internal monitoring is more accurate than external monitoring, but it does

have some drawbacks. Your baby may run the risk of contracting an infection from the electrode attached to her scalp; and the use of the monitor restricts your mobility, which may slow down the progress of your labour. Because of these factors, internal monitoring is normally only carried out when there are proven benefits to the mother or baby.

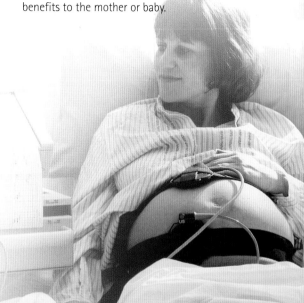

PAIN RELIEF

If you're feeling apprehensive about how you'll cope during labour, don't worry, you're not alone. Every pregnant woman has the same fears and yet, one way or another, we all get through it and are usually prepared to endure it again! No pain is pleasant, but consider labour pain as a 'positive pain' – you know there is a beginning and an end, after which you will have your beautiful, longed-for baby.

Although there is no way of gauging how intense your contractions will be or how you will manage with the pain, your attitude can help you enormously. Fear and anxiety will make you more tense and less able to cope, whereas the more in control and calm you feel, the more you will be able to 'ride' with the pain. Be open-minded about what you might need and don't put yourself through pain unnecessarily: it will leave you more exhausted, just at the time when you'll need all your energy to care for your new baby.

Natural pain relief

Over the centuries, women have used a variety of techniques to make labour more comfortable and medical intervention less likely. If successful, you may find you need fewer or no pain-killing drugs. Certain breathing and postural techniques may be sufficient to deal with any discomfort. However, there also are other natural methods of pain management to try, including the meditation on page 278, none of which will have any side effects on you or your baby.

Breathing
In early labour, slow breathing helps to promote and maintain relaxation. Taking deep, relaxing breaths at the beginning and end of contractions enhances the

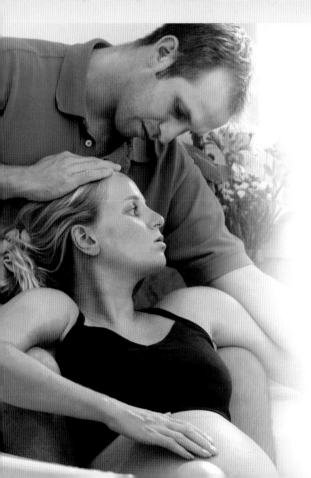

delivery of oxygen. When you breathe, try not to panic and hyperventilate (breathe too quickly), and don't hold your breath for prolonged periods.

The mental effort required to slow down breathing and relax muscles can also serve as a distraction from painful contractions. Relaxed muscles make it much easier for your uterus to do its work so that they are also more likely to stretch as your baby passes through your pelvis.

In late labour, if the descent of your baby triggers the urge to push before your cervix is fully dilated, your healthcare provider may recommend panting or deep blowing, as if you're trying to keep a feather floating. This type of breathing also is helpful if you need to slow down pushing at the time of actual delivery of your baby's head. Breathing out stops your lungs from expanding and pushing down on your uterus at a time when pushing isn't appropriate.

Birthing pools

Even if you don't want to give birth in the pool, sitting immersed in warm, soothing water can bring relief during contractions. Ask if your hospital has one; if not, they can be hired.

Massage

Kneading or stroking muscles can help to release muscle tension and promote relaxation. Relaxation, in turn, can increase blood circulation to muscles, helping to ensure that they have adequate oxygen. Between contractions, massage can provide a pleasant tactile sensation to help to lift your spirits, while during contractions massage can help to take your mind off the pain.

Typically, most women want to be massaged during the first stage and for strokes to become stronger and more frequent as contractions get stronger.

If you're suffering from lower back pain, you may like to ask your birth partner to gently rub the area, particularly around the sacrum (where your spine joins your pelvis). He should make a series of large circles using the heel of his hands followed by smaller circles made with the thumbs. Your partner also can apply stronger sacral pressure by placing one hand on top of the other, criss-cross fashion, pressing from the level of the hips down to the coccyx.

Acupuncture

This can be used at the start of contractions and throughout labour. Fine, sterilised needles are inserted into points along invisible channels or meridians in the body. The Chinese believe that good health depends upon the flow of 'chi' or energy along these channels. Backache during labour, for instance, may occur as a result of a blockage along the meridians. The needles are used to release such blockages so that 'chi' energy can flow freely.

TENS machines

These send a small electrical current, which blocks the pain impulses to the brain and also stimulates the release of endorphins, your body's own natural painkillers. Many hospitals have TENS machines, or they can be hired.

Hypnosis

Sessions during the latter stages of pregnancy can store positive, relieving images in the subconscious mind, which can later be brought to the fore when you need them, helping you through labour.

Positions

When it comes to giving birth, an upright position is best, as it enlists the aid of gravity to help to push your baby out. You may want to stick to one position or try out a few; do whatever makes you feel most comfortable. Try squatting against your birth partner or a wall; kneeling forward on a pile of cushions or sitting upright against them; or kneeling upright with support. There may be times when you need to sit or lie down to get comfortable. Try sitting on a chair the wrong way around, so you're facing the chair back; going on all-fours if you are experiencing backache, or lying on your side on the floor, resting on pillows.

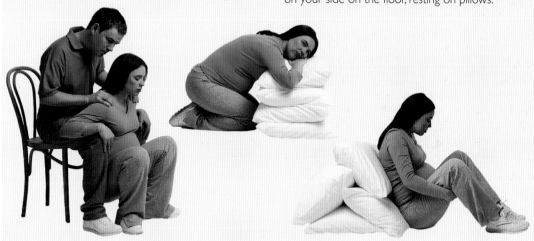

Find relief from pain

Use this meditation when you want to

- Practise controlling your breathing in preparation for labour

- Cope as effectively as possible with pain during delivery

How to practise this meditation

You will find that the breathing techniques and ways of focusing your mind used during meditation will be helpful in keeping you calm and in control during your labour. Bear in mind that the first stage of labour can last many hours, so try to pace yourself.

As each contraction builds up, feeling like a tight band around your abdomen, concentrate on your breathing, taking deep breaths and keeping it slow and controlled. It will help if you can keep in mind a relaxing image or to focus on an object in the room – something you've brought that you have used as a calming visual aid in the past, or even just the end of the bed. As the contraction begins to fade, consciously relax your shoulders and let your body relax in preparation for the next one. Silently repeat a mantra or affirmation which will help to give you confidence to keep going, such as.

- One contraction more is one contraction less
- I am coping
- It comes, it goes
- There is an end

As labour progresses, keep in mind all the things you've learned over the past few months to prepare you for this wonderful event. Focus your mind, use your partner for emotional and physical support, and find the position in which you feel most comfortable.

Medical pain relief

It's very important to think about what type of pain relief you might want during labour, as your choice can make a big difference to your birth experience. Keep an open mind, so that you remain flexible and tuned in to your actual labour experience. Among the standard medical therapies are analgesics, which relieve pain, anaesthetics, which block sensations, and tranquilizers, which calm you. Local anaesthetic can be given at the time of birth. Local anaesthetics are commonly used for epidural insertion, episiotomies and pudendal blocks.

Analgesics

Drugs that are injected into a muscle or given intravenously, analgesics dull pain and can make you sleepy if they're narcotic based. Pethidine is the most common analgesic used in labour, and is given either by injection in the buttocks or intravenously when labour is established. It can be particularly helpful when early labour is prolonged and uncomfortable, helping you to rest and taking the edge off strong sensations. It can make you drowsy, which may help you to cope with the passage of time in labour.

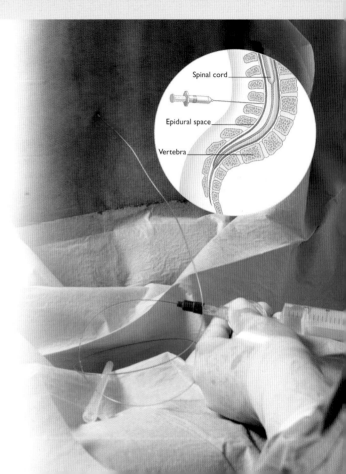

Spinal cord

Epidural space

Vertebra

On the negative side, analgesics can hinder your ability to get up and walk about during labour, because they can make you unsteady on your feet. Also, you may dislike feeling drowsy and out of control. If given close to delivery, pethidine can make your baby drowsy and slow to feed and interact. It also may impair his breathing and he may need extra oxygen. The effects on your baby can last longer than they do on you, as his immature system is less capable of clearing the medication from his body. Medication can be given to the baby after birth to reverse these effects.

Epidural

This regional anaesthetic is the most popular choice for pain relief during labour. An epidural blocks most pain sensations in the abdomen, although you can still feel pressure. Only an anaesthetist, a specialist in anaesthesia, can administer an epidural. This is done by placing a small needle into the epidural space, in the lower part of your back. The needle passes between the bones of the lower vertebrae, below the location of the spinal cord. A very tiny, sterile tube is threaded through the needle. The needle is then removed, leaving the tiny tube in place. Medications are given through the tube, including narcotics to take away pain and sometimes local anaesthetic drugs that block pain but cause numbness. Once the medication is injected into the tube, you may feel relief from any pain in ten minutes.

Epidural medication can be injected into the epidural tube either by periodic injections or by connecting the tube to a pump. Whereas injections tend to wear off after some time, a pump is designed to provide a continuous low dose of the drug.

When epidurals include a local anaesthetic drug, which causes numbness, you may experience little or no feeling, which means that it can be difficult to urinate. A small catheter or tube will be inserted through the urethra into the bladder so that it can be emptied. An epidural may also make it difficult to push at the end of labour. Sitting in a relatively upright position for delivery – at a 45- to 90-degree angle – and concentrating on pushing can help.

Epidurals also can lower your blood pressure. Since it is essential to keep your circulation going so that your baby gets enough oxygen, your blood pressure will be monitored frequently before and after an epidural is inserted. In addition, you'll be given fluids via an IV to keep your circulating blood volume stable. Your baby will be monitored by an electronic fetal monitor.

While some women complain of backache after birth, it is more likely that this comes from the inability to move around a lot in labour and the passage of the baby through the pelvis. Research has found no link between epidurals and long-term lower back pain. Some women do, however, experience headaches after an epidural. This happens if there is a leak of spinal fluid after the epidural is inserted. If the headache persists, it can be treated with a 'blood patch', which involves a small amount of blood being taken from a vein on the woman's arm, and injecting it into the epidural space, sealing the leak.

Pudendal block

Another type of regional anaesthetic this is given at the time of delivery, by a needle inserted through the vagina. As these anaesthetics numb only this perineal area, you'll feel less pain, but you'll still feel contractions. It's usually given with forceps or vacuum extraction and its effect can last through an episiotomy and subsequent stitching.

Tranquillisers

These are muscle relaxants, which can relieve tension. They are usually given with a narcotic to maximize the effect of a small dose of narcotic.

General anaesthesia

This is anaesthetic gas mixed with oxygen and is only given if medically necessary, in particular during an emergency Caesarean. When you awake, you may feel drowsy. It may have the same sedative effect on your baby. Giving a general anaesthetic as close to the birth as possible will help to minimize any effect it may have on your baby.

THE STAGES OF CHILDBIRTH

Childbirth is divided into three stages. During the first stage of labour, uterine contractions work to fully dilate or open out the cervix. The second, or pushing, stage is the time it takes for your baby to pass out of the uterus, squeeze down the birth canal and out into the outside world. The third stage is the delivery of the placenta. During your baby's journey down the 23-cm long birth canal (the seamless connection of uterus, cervix and vagina) , he will change position, completing a 90˚ rotation. He will turn again once his head is born. Your baby assists with his birth by pushing himself away from your uterine wall with his feet and by wriggling his head through your cervix.

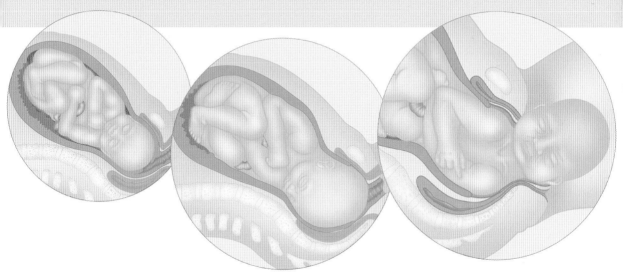

The first stage

The first stage of labour, is often divided into three phases: early or latent labour, active labour and transition or hard labour. For many women, these stages are distinct and noticeable. Other women may not notice such clear-cut differences.

Early or latent labour

This is usually the longest but easiest stage. During this time, the cervix continues to thin out and progressively dilates to 3 or 4 cm. At this stage, you may be aware of contractions, but they're usually manageable, and you may be able to sleep through them.

Contractions are usually short, lasting from 20 to 60 seconds. Initially they may be as far apart as 20 minutes, becoming increasingly stronger and closer over a six- to eight-hour period. This may be the point at which the mucus plug is dislodged or your membranes rupture.

Your symptoms in early labour may be similar to those of pre-labour – cramps, backache, increased urination and bowel movements, increased vaginal discharge, pelvic pressure, and leg and hip cramps.

What to do in early labour

- Unless there's a medical reason for you to go early to the hospital, you'll be much more comfortable staying at home in early labour.
- If you first notice the contractions at night, continue resting as much as possible. If you can't rest, find a distracting, but not taxing, activity. Don't forget to eat light snacks during this early stage. Eating light solids in labour can actually improve labour outcome – labour is hard work and your body needs energy in order to cope.

Many women also experience a burst of energy, but try to conserve this energy for later on.

Active labour

This Is reached when the cervix begins to dilate rapidly. For first-time mothers in this stage, the cervix usually dilates at a minimum of 1 cm an hour. Contractions become noticeably more intense, and if a cervical check is performed, you'll probably be 3 cm dilated. Contractions now last 45 to 60 seconds, getting progressively stronger and closer together, from occurring about every five to seven minutes to every two to three minutes.

Contractions will feel a lot stronger now, and you may experience increased aches and tiredness. Your membranes may rupture if they haven't already. You'll probably feel a lot less sociable now as you focus in on yourself.

What to do in active labour

- As contractions become stronger and longer, you may need to work harder to relax through and between contractions. Try moving around and changing your position to relieve muscle tension. The sheer physical effort of labour can lead to increased breathing, heart rate, perspiration and even nausea. It's important to drink plenty of cool liquids to guard against dehydration.
- Women in this stage of labour sometimes feel that labour is never going to end. Try to remember that this phase is usually rapid and the cervix will be dilated soon. You also may worry about how well things are progressing, so ask your healthcare provider about anything that's bothering you. If you find this difficult for any reason, you may prefer your birth partner to ask on your behalf.

Transitional labour

Lasting between around one and two hours, transition is labour's most difficult and demanding period, during which the cervix fully dilates from 8 to 10 cm. Contractions now become very strong, lasting from 60 to 90 seconds and coming every two to three minutes. Where you might have made rapid progress through the active phase, everything can seem to slow down during transitional labour. Be assured, however, that the end is in sight.

Because of the intensity of this phase, dramatic physical and emotional changes can accompany it. As your baby is pushed into your pelvis, you'll experience strong pressure in your lower back and/or perineum. You may have the urge to push or move your bowels and your legs may become shaky and weak. Significant stress reactions aren't uncommon, with perspiration, hyperventilation, shivering, nausea, vomiting and exhaustion all possible. Without meaning to, women can reject the help of their birth partners and find every touch or labour aid unacceptable during this phase.

Many women lose all inhibitions, and even may verbalise their distress uncharacteristically by shouting and swearing.

What to do during transition

- Keep the goal in sight. The pushing stage will come soon and your discomfort will be much more controllable. Bear in mind that stronger contractions bring the phase to an end faster.
- Don't be afraid to express yourself – make it clear what helps and what doesn't. Try also to relax; it's the key to conserving strength and the best way to help contractions to accomplish their goal.

The second stage

Once you are through the transition period the time has come to push your baby out. The second stage usually takes an hour, but can take as little as ten minutes or as much as three hours. As with early labour, the second stage may be significantly lengthened if anaesthesia has been given.

Even after a long, exhausting labour, many women find a renewed burst of energy in the second stage, as they've achieved full dilation of the cervix and know that birth is imminent. Now you can take a much more active and mentally distracting role, which can make you feel a lot more positive.

The second stage can have another significant plus: bearing down with contractions can make discomfort seem to disappear. As long as the second stage isn't too fast and allows the perineum to stretch gradually, it can be a time of pressure, not pain. Often the extreme pressure of the baby's tight fit and the subsequent compression of nerves leads to a form of anaesthesia itself. For many women, this nerve compression blocks the sensation of perineal tears or an episiotomy (see page 293).

Contractions in the second stage still last for 60 to 90 seconds but may come every two to four minutes. Your position can influence their pattern – staying upright can intensify contractions; reclining and knee-chest positions may slow them down.

What to do in the second stage

- You'll have an overwhelming urge to push, but it's important to wait until your healthcare provider says that it's okay. You'll feel huge pressure on your rectum, and a tingling, burning feeling as your baby's head appears at the entrance to your vagina. Your emotions may veer now from exhaustion and tearfulness to excitement at the thought of meeting your baby at last.

The third stage

Once your baby is born, the placenta is delivered, which ensures the complete removal of the pregnancy. For most deliveries, this is relatively automatic and requires little effort. In fact, you may be so involved with your baby that you don't pay much attention to the procedure. Most units , however, recommend active management of the third stage of labour to prevent heavy bleeding after delivery.

As soon as your baby leaves your uterus, the uterus continues to contract, causing a massive decrease in volume, which usually shears the less flexible placenta from its walls. Further contractions push the placenta out. Immediately after the baby is born, an injection of syntocinon (synthetic oxytocin) or syntometrine is given into your upper leg, which encourages the uterus to stay contracted. This allows the birth attendant to help the placenta to be expelled by gently pulling on the cord. If you're lying down, he or she may massage your uterus or ask you to bear down and push.

Early breastfeeding helps to prevent problems with bleeding from the site of the placenta, as nipple stimulation releases oxytocin, the hormone that

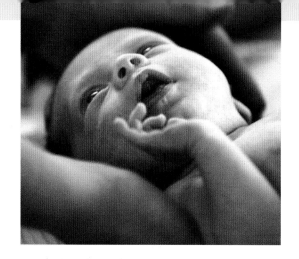

promotes uterine contractions. If you have increased bleeding, your doctor may give you syntocinon via an IV, to help the uterus to contract and decrease postnatal bleeding. Once the placenta is out, it will be examined to check that fragments haven't broken off inside the uterus. Very occasionally retained placenta occurs, when the placenta remains behind in the uterus. To remove it, an obstetrician needs to feel inside the uterus and manually remove it. This usually takes place in the operating room under epidural.

Induction

Left to nature, most women will go into labour and deliver their babies within two weeks either side of their due date. Labour is induced when it's better for the baby to be born than remain inside the uterus or when the health of mother or baby is deemed at risk should the pregnancy continue.

If a baby isn't growing sufficiently towards the end of a pregnancy or has a serious medical condition, ending a pregnancy by inducing labour may be the best option. Mothers who have high-risk conditions, such as diabetes or pregnancy-induced hypertension, may be candidates for induction. Even if your labour is not induced, your healthcare provider may help the progress of labour by using syntocinon (a synthetic form of oxytocin) to make your contractions stronger and more effective.

Syntocinon should be given in such a way as to simulate normal contractions. However, artificially induced contractions are often stronger and more frequent than natural contractions. This, in turn, can lead to abnormal fetal heart readings, so women who are receiving syntocinon are almost always on a fetal monitor to see how the baby is tolerating the contractions. If the frequency of contractions is too high, the dose may be adjusted downwards.

Elective induction

Some doctors and women prefer to 'plan' delivery and will schedule a date for the mother to be induced at the end of her pregnancy. Before beginning an induction, particularly an elective induction, the healthcare provider must assure that delivery is the best option for the baby, and there are special tests that can be performed to check if the baby is 'ready'.

In cases of elective inductions, the baby should be at full term. Delivering a baby electively too early – such as three weeks before the due date – may put the newborn at risk.

Forceps and ventouse

These medical instruments are used to help to ease the baby out of the birth canal. Studies show that certain medications and positions in labour may increase the likelihood that these will need to be used. It's wise to talk to your healthcare provider about his or her thoughts on the use of both forceps and vacuum extractors long before you go into labour.

Forceps

Metal instruments resembling salad tongs or spoons may be used if the mother can't push effectively or if the baby has to be born quickly. The use of forceps may prevent the need for a Caesarean birth. Forceps also can be used to turn the baby into a different position and, while forceps can cause more damage to the perineum, they can reduce the chances of trauma to the baby.

Opponents of forceps maintain that they can be used out of convenience when labour is slow and the medical team want the baby to be delivered as quickly as possible.

Ventouse or vacuum extractor

This works in a similar way to forceps, but instead of metal tongs, a soft suction cup is placed on the baby's head. Suction helps to pull the baby out as the mother pushes. Vacuum extractors can be used higher up the birth canal than forceps and cause less damage to the perineum.

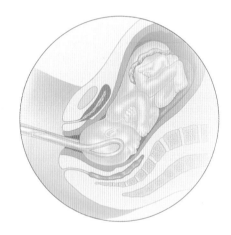

Episiotomy

This is a small cut made in the perineum (the skin between the vagina and anus) in order to enlarge the vaginal opening when the baby's head is about to be born. The favoured incision is the mediolateral, where the cut is angled a little to one side, away from the rectum. Although it is harder to repair and causes more blood loss than cutting straight down (a midline incision), it has the advantage of greater protection of the integrity of the rectum.

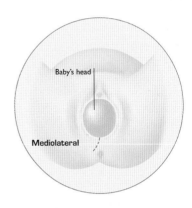

In many hospitals, episiotomies used to be performed routinely. However, over the last two decades there has been a significant reduction in the percentage of deliveries involving episiotomies and the current thinking is that there's no absolute benefit of routine episiotomies. Frequently, the skill and patience of an experienced healthcare provider will stretch the area and allow the baby to be born with minimal or no tears and no episiotomy. Sometimes a small tear is easily repaired and causes less pain than a large and invasive episiotomy.

Episiotomy is still considered valuable in a few situations, for instance when forceps or ventouse are employed, if the perineum hasn't stretched sufficiently during the pushing stage, to shorten the pushing stage because of fetal distress, if the baby's head is too large or if the mother has a medical problem such as a heart condition and cannot cope with a long labour. An episiotomy may be recommended to protect the delicate skull of a premature infant or to provide more space for the delivery of breech or very large babies.

Caesarean sections

Most Caesareans are performed for medical reasons and are planned for in advance. An emergency Caesarean may be performed when a serious medical condition, such as pre-eclampsia (see page 239) makes rapid delivery necessary. While some women might prefer to have a Caesarean birth to avoid the discomfort of labour, it is not recommended nor acceptable practice. Only an obstetrician or a surgeon can perform a Caesarean, and although surgical techniques have improved vastly in recent years, there are still much greater risks associated with Caesareans than with vaginal births. In addition, the recovery period can be considerably longer, and a Caesarean may make subsequent vaginal births more difficult.

While Caesareans can be a safer means of birth for some babies - those at risk of trauma from the birth process such as extremely premature babies or those in distress – there are effects that may need to be overcome. Sometimes Caesarean babies can retain fluid in their lungs – this is normally squeezed out in the birth canal. The newborn also may be drowsy from medication given to the mother.

Recognized reasons for a caesarean

- If the baby is in a difficult position for delivery - breech position (feet or buttocks first) or transverse (lying sideways in the uterus).
- If the baby is very large.
- If the mother has a high-risk condition, such as bleeding, genital herpes, diabetes and pregnancy-induced hypertension or eclampsia (see page 240).
- If there's more than one baby.
- If the baby is not growing well, has a high-risk condition or is suffering fetal distress as a result of the stresses and strains of labour.

A typical procedure

Depending on your medical condition and the reason for the Caesarean, you'll be given either a general or a regional anaesthetic. A catheter (a small tube) will be placed in your bladder to drain urine during your Caesarean and for several hours following surgery. Your abdomen will be prepared with an antiseptic wash and sterile drapes; a small area will be shaved for the incision, which will be made with a scalpel through the skin in the lower abdomen. The muscles of the abdomen aren't usually cut but are separated in the midline and pushed aside. The bladder may be pushed down to protect it from instruments. Another incision will be made in the uterus. You may hear a whooshing noise as the amniotic fluid is sucked out.

Once your uterus is open, your baby will be lifted out through the incision. Frequently at this time, the top of the uterus is squeezed – just as you would do when pushing – and you'll feel pressure and a tugging sensation. The baby will be handed to another member of the team, who will examine her and perform some basic tests. You may be able to see your baby immediately or after she has been assessed physically.

After the doctor has removed the placenta, your uterus and the layers of the abdominal wall will be sewn closed with absorbable sutures. Your skin will then be closed with either sutures or staples. Once this is done, you will probably be united with your baby before you leave the surgical suite for the recovery unit.

Your new baby

Congratulations – at last you have your long-awaited baby! The anticipation of the last nine months is over, the daunting prospect of labour has come and gone and now you can concentrate all your energies on your precious infant. Although you are probably feeling exhausted, the excitement of having a new addition to the family and caring for this small, vulnerable being will somehow carry you through the fatigue of the early weeks. But get as much rest as you can and give yourself time to recover by accepting any help offered. Fit in your meditations when you can, if only for a few minutes each day, and use the time to relax and focus on getting your body back to optimum health.

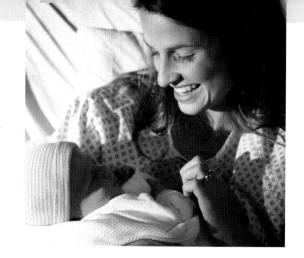

Holding your newborn in your arms for the first time is a truly amazing and emotional experience. The intense love a mother feels for her child is like no other and is something to be cherished. The bonding process, however, can take longer to set in for some women than for others, so don't panic if you don't feel immediate love. The awesome responsibility of looking after something so small, needy and vulnerable, however, hits all new mothers (and fathers).

Don't forget that your emotions – heightened by the physical experience of delivery, the exhaustion that comes with sleepless nights and a demanding baby – will probably be swinging all over the place. Meditating during these early weeks can not only help to centre you but also provide you with a few rare minutes to yourself. Even if you can't closet yourself away physically, you can mentally withdraw to a more peaceful place while you are doing something else, such as breast-feeding or changing your baby's nappy.

Immediate baby needs

Breastfeeding
- ❏ Breast pads – non-plastic backed

If expressing:
- ❏ Pump
- ❏ 2 bottles and teats
- ❏ Sterilizing tablets or sterilizer
- ❏ Bottlebrush

Bottlefeeding
- ❏ 6 bottles and teats
- ❏ Sterilizer
- ❏ Bottlebrush
- ❏ Bottle warmer – optional

Changing
- ❏ Changing mat/table
- ❏ Baby wipes
- ❏ Cotton wool
- ❏ 70 first-size disposable nappies
- ❏ Nappy sacks

Or
- ❏ 24 cloth nappies
- ❏ Safety pins or clips
- ❏ Plastic pants
- ❏ 2 nappy buckets
- ❏ Sterilizing fluid
- ❏ Nappy liners

Clothes
- ❏ 4 babygrows
- ❏ 2 nightdresses or sleep suits or 2 extra babygrows
- ❏ 4 cotton vests
- ❏ 3 cardigans
- ❏ 2 bibs
- ❏ 2 shawls
- ❏ Hat – type depending on season
- ❏ Mittens

Bedtime
- ❏ Moses basket or cradle or cot and cot mattress
- ❏ 3 fitted bottom sheets
- ❏ 3 top sheets – optional
- ❏ 2 or 3 lightweight blankets

Bathing
- ❏ Baby bath
- ❏ Cotton wool
- ❏ Mild baby shampoo
- ❏ 2 large soft towels
- ❏ Flannel or sponge
- ❏ Baby hairbrush
- ❏ Blunt-ended scissors

Celebrate the birth

Use this meditation when you want to

- Welcome the newest member of your family

- Give thanks for your baby's safe delivery

- Cope with being overwhelmed by your feelings for your newborn

How to practise this meditation

For the first few days after the birth of your baby, you will probably find it easiest to fit in a few mini meditations. Use the time to focus your thoughts and energies, starting off by just becoming aware of your breathing. Focus on the flow of your breath as it enters and leaves your nose, cool on the inhalation and warm on the exhalation. Feel your shoulders relax down and notice how all the tension in your body flows out from your head to your toes.

If you are feeling overwhelmed by emotions for your newborn, you may prefer to spend your precious few minutes of meditation concentrating on something other than your baby. In this case, try focusing on a tree, a vase of flowers, or a mandala instead.

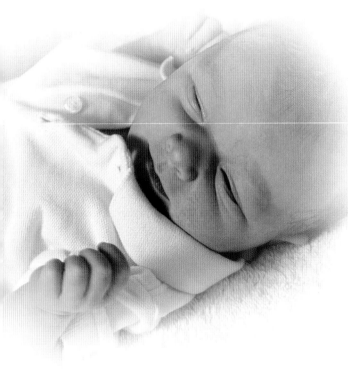

If, however, you want your baby to be the focus for your meditation, choose a mantra or affirmation which reflects the way you feel. You can either devise your own, or try one of the following:

- We are one
- Om
- Love
- My longed for baby is here
- I give thanks for my baby
- Love encompasses all

Say the mantra or affirmation out loud so that your newborn hears the comforting sound of your voice.

Index

C

D

E

Acknowledgements

Picture credits

85 Zephyr/Science Photo Library
147 Mother & Baby PL/Ian Hooton
160 Photolibrary Group
176-177 Photolibrary Group
202 Spa Village, Pangkor Laut Resort, Malaysia
215 Photolibrary Group
222 Photolibrary Group
243 Mother & Baby PL/Ruth Jenkinson
268 Ian Hooton/Science Photo Library
273 Mother & Baby PL/Ruth Jenkinson
280 Photolibrary Group

Illustrations

Halli Marie Verrinder
Amanda Williams

Useful addresses

Well Mother www.wellmother.org
TAMBA (Twins and Multiple Births Association)
www.tamba.org.uk
3 Steps to Fertility www.3stepstofertility.co.uk

Related Carroll & Brown books

3 Steps to Fertility Marina Nicholas
Fertility and Conception Dr. Karen Trewinnard
Your Pregnancy Bible by Dr. Anne Deans
Your Pregnancy Day-by-Day by Professor
Stuart Campbell
The Complete Pregnancy Cookbook by Fiona Wilcock
Watch Me Grow by Professor Stuart Campbell
Pregnancy Exercise by Judy Di Fiore
Natural Pregnancy by Susannah Marriott
Caesarean Recovery by Chrissie Gallagher-Mundy
Beautiful Birth by Suzanne Yates
Instinctive Birthing by Val Clarke
Babycare by Dr. Frances Williams
Baby Massage by Peter Walker
Baby Fun by Annette Knecht-Boyer
A Dad's Guide to Babycare by Colin Cooper
The Wonder Years by Dr. Martin Ward Platt
Understanding Your Crying Baby by Sheila Kitzinger